Child health matters

Child health matters

Caring for children in the community

Edited by Sally Wyke and Jenny Hewison

Open University Press
Milton Keynes · Philadelphia

Open University Press
Celtic Court
22 Ballmoor
Buckingham MK18 1XW

and
1900 Frost Road, Suite 101
Bristol, PA 19007, USA

First Published 1991

British Library Cataloguing in Publication Data

Child health matters: caring for children in the community.
   1. Great Britain. Community health services for children
I. Wyke, Sally   II. Hewison, Jenny
362.19892000941

ISBN 0 335 09394 9
    0 335 09393 0 (pbk)

Library of Congress Cataloging-in-Publication Data

Child health matters: caring for children in the community/
   edited by Sally Wyke and Jenny Hewison.
      p.   cm.
   Includes index.
   ISBN 0-335-09394-9 (hardback) — ISBN 0-335-09393-0 (pbk.)
   1. Community health services for children. I. Wyke, Sally, 1959–   .
   II. Hewison, Jenny, 1950–   .
   RJ101.C5254   1990
   362.1'9892—dc20
                                      90-14259 CIP

Typeset by Scarborough Typesetting Services
Printed in Great Britain by St Edmundsbury Press
Bury St Edmunds, Suffolk

For
Bill and Ben
Robert and Katie

Contents

viii   Contents

Notes on contributors

Andy Clarke has a Psychology degree from Stirling University. He has a longstanding interest in the politics of racial equality. In 1985, he went to work with Jenny Hewison in the Leeds University Psychology Department, conducting research for a PhD concerning how parents in multi-ethnic areas use general practitioner services on behalf of their children. Andy has given a number of conference papers and seminars about his work, and he is currently preparing articles based on his thesis for publication in medical and social science journals.

Sarah Cunningham-Burley is a lecturer in Medical Sociology at the Department of Community Medicine, University of Dundee. Her research interests broadly focus on the family and health, and on qualitative methods. Previously, she has worked as research sociologist at the Medical Research Council's Medical Sociology Unit, Glasgow, where she conducted two studies, the first on 'Marital Status and Pregnancy Outcome' and the second on 'Health Education for Young Teenagers and their Knowledge of AIDS'. She is co-editor (with Neil McKeganey) of two books: *Enter the Sociologist: Reflections on the Practice of Sociology* (Avebury, 1987) and *Readings on Medical Sociology* (Routledge, 1990).

Caroline Currer qualified as a psychiatric social worker in 1971 and spent the next 7 years working in a mental health centre in north-west Pakistan. She worked with mentally ill Pathan people, especially women and their families, helped to set up a training centre for mentally handicapped children, and collaborated in a research project to investigate the extent of psychiatric disorder in a rural area. The first of her three children was born in Pakistan, and this has been a significant factor in her subsequent interest in migrant mothering. Since 1979 she has been based at the University of Warwick. She has conducted research funded by the DHSS concerning the mental health of Pathan women, and their views of maternity and child health services, and went on to investigate services for mentally handicapped people and their families in north Warwickshire. From 1986 to 1989 she taught the Sociology of Health and Healing at undergraduate and postgraduate levels. She is co-editor (with Meg Stacey) of *Concepts of Health, Illness and Disease: A Comparative Perspective* (Berg, 1986).

Robert Drewett worked initially as a research fellow of the Population Council, and is now a Lecturer in Psychology at Durham University. His interests are in medical applications of psychology, and he has worked with paediatricians and midwives on the problems of human lactation. These collaborations have included numerous research studies in the UK, as well as a large-scale field study of nursing and weaning in relation to child growth and health in rural Thailand. Robert Drewett has published widely in journals and books devoted to child development, health and nutrition.

Heather Fletcher is a consultant community paediatrician in Northumberland. Some of her Senior Registrar training was based in North Tyneside where two major studies on childhood asthma have been conducted. Her major research was a survey of childhood asthma deaths in the Northern Region (1970–85). Much of her clinical work is concerned with children in vulnerable families and those who have experience of abuse, deprivation and family disruption.

Jenny Hewison has a degree in Natural Sciences from Cambridge University. After several years as a full-time researcher in London and Newcastle upon Tyne, she is now a Lecturer in Psychology at the University of Leeds. Her research interests are in applied areas of health, education and child development. She is currently working on a study of the quality of care which general practitioners provide for children, and a study of the ways in which mothers reconcile family and employment obligations when their children are ill. Jenny has one daughter.

Jenny Kitzinger graduated in Social Anthropology from Cambridge University. She has worked as a researcher in the Child Care and Development Unit at Cambridge and is now based in the Sociology Department of Glasgow University. Her current paid work is on AIDS and the media. She was involved in setting up the Cambridge Incest Survivors Refuge where she worked as a volunteer for several years. She has run training workshops on child sexual abuse for various professional groups and her work on sexual violence has appeared in a range of books and journals aimed at health practitioners as well as lay and academic audiences. Jenny is presently writing a book about surviving sexual violence, to be published by Pandora Press in 1991.

Una Maclean is a Reader in Community Medicine at Edinburgh University. Her research, in Africa and in Scotland, has combined epidemiology and ethnomedicine. She is the author of five books and numerous articles. Cancer epidemiology in Nigeria led her to a study of Yoruba traditional medicine, with special reference to women's health-related behaviour. Since then, her central concern has been with women's health and studies have included a psychiatric survey in the Outer Hebrides of Scotland; an exploration of how women respond to men's heart attacks; women's reasons for declining breast screening; the domestic dilemmas of poor mothers in a deprived urban housing estate; mothers' monitoring of young children's symptoms; and the burdens on women as community carers of the frail and elderly. The emphasis throughout has been on the unique interpretations that women place upon symptoms and personal misfortunes and the frequent lack of fit between their views and those of care providers. Dr Maclean is widowed, with five children.

Berry Mayall has worked at the Thomas Coram Research Unit for 16 years on a range of research studies. A particular focus of her work has been on day-care provision for the under-fives. During the last 8 years her work has been funded under the ESRC's Designated Research Scheme and she has planned and carried out a programme of work on child health care. She has published extensively from this work, including: (with Pat Petrie) *Childminding and Day-nurseries – What Kind of Care?* (Heinemann Educational, 1983); *Keeping Children Healthy* (Allen and Unwin, 1986); (with Marie-Claude Foster) *Child Health Care: Living with Children, Working for Children* (Heinemann, 1989).

Jacqueline Mok graduated from Edinburgh University Medical School in 1974, and is at present a Consultant Paediatrician in Community Child Health with the Lothian Health Board. She has responsibility for the integration and care of children with chronic diseases and handicap in the community, liaising with social work departments as well as the Department of Education. Since January 1986, her special interest has been in the care and follow-up of infants at risk of HIV infection. Edinburgh has a particular problem with the numbers of young women infected with HIV, and Dr Mok has the largest cohort of infants born to HIV-infected women in the UK. Her personal research interests are to evaluate the risk of mother-to-child transmission of HIV and to define the natural history of perinatally acquired HIV disease. Therapeutic regimes are also being tried on children who present with signs and symptoms of HIV disease.

Jennie Popay is a social policy analyst. She worked as a teacher of geomorphology in Lancashire and Africa for a number of years before completing her first degree in New Zealand. On moving back to Britain, she shifted her focus to health and social policy, and completed a Master's degree at Essex University in 1977. Since then, she has conducted a number of research projects concerning: inequalities in health related to social class;

gender and ethnicity; the policy implications of changes in family life and patterns of employment; and the social and economic costs of unemployment and the recession. She has published numerous articles and book chapters in all of these areas. During 1983–5, she worked on the Open University Course 'Health and Disease', a unique multidisciplinary approach to the field of health, illness and social policy. Jennie is currently Senior Research Officer at the University of London's Thomas Coram Research Institute, where her current research concerns patterns of health and health care in families with dependent children and the relationship between paid and domestic labour and adult health.

Ian Russell was educated at Cambridge, Birmingham and Essex universities. Since 1987, he has been Director of the new Health Services Research Unit at Aberdeen University, concentrating on the effectiveness and efficiency of hospital services. For 17 years before that, he worked at the Health Care Research Unit of Newcastle University, concentrating on the quality of care in general practice. He has also held visiting appointments at the universities of Keele, North Carolina, York and the United States National Institute of Environmental Health Sciences.

Elizabeth Watson is Research Fellow in the Department of Clinical Epidemiology, London Hospital Medical College, and has been engaged in research in the inner city since 1975. She is a member of the Council of Management and of the Support and Information Committee of the Foundation for Study of Infant Deaths. She has published numerous papers on the sudden infant death syndrome, post-neonatal mortality, health visiting, the health of different ethnic groups in the inner city, and evaluation in the child health services.

Sally Wyke graduated in Human Sciences from University College London in 1982. She then moved to the Health Care Research Unit, University of Newcastle upon Tyne, where she was attached to the first British study of standards and performance in general practice. Here she conducted research for her PhD concerning parents' consulting behaviour for their child's respiratory illness and has written a number of articles based on this research. Since completing her PhD, she was worked on a longitudinal study of elderly people at the University College of North Wales, and is presently Research Fellow at the Medical Research Council's Medical Sociology Unit in Glasgow, where she is working on a longitudinal study of the social patterning of health and illness. Sally's research interests include: inequalities in health through the life-cycle; associations between economic status and health; and health service utilization. She has a longstanding commitment to making her research accessible to practitioners and planners who may find the results useful.

Preface

This book is timely because it cannot have escaped the reader's notice that the Health Services are under review. Sweeping changes in management arrangements are to be introduced which will undoubtedly change how the services are offered. The White Paper on the Health Service gives its overall objective as: for patients, better health care and greater choice of the services available; for staff, greater satisfaction and rewards for those working in the NHS who successfully respond to local needs and preferences. It is for the District Health Authorities to ensure that the health needs of the population for which they are responsible are met. What might they be?

One high objective is that as many children as possible reach adulthood with their potential uncompromised by illness or environmental hazard. The best way of achieving that end would be to enable parents to do as much of the care as possible themselves. How can we in the health care services help? Many of the chapters in this book report research and introduce the reader to the literature which is directed at that question.

If we are to ask just *what is needed* then perhaps the most appropriate people to ask would be the mothers of young children. They would of course have to know what is possible and what is available. That poses another problem. *What is best* for the children as far as their health is concerned? Do parents know what is best? Goldstein, Freud and Solnit in 'Beyond the Best Interests of the Child' state as a conviction that parents should generally be entitled to raise their children as they think best, free from state intervention. Does the Health Authority know what is best for the children's health? Do the doctors? Do the Health Visitors? These are not easy matters but they need to be addressed. Many of the chapters you will read touch on the responsibilities of professionals and how they are viewed by parents, particularly mothers. Health visiting and the child health and school medical services were established to help those children who, for whatever reason, were not being cared for adequately by their parents. Those services still have that responsibility.

There is the risk that what the *children need* might be interpreted as what the parents want, or what the health professionals want. Again, we need to make fine distinctions. Not only are parents the people who usually decide what they want for their children, they also provide most of the care. So what they want in order to provide that care is a critical question. The message that is clear in many of these chapters is that the answer depends on the strengths, characteristics and beliefs of the family, particularly the mother. We would surely want a service for children which does not share equally but shares according to need. Mothers from different cultures have different expectations and different ways of coping; I hope we would wish to provide a service which is equally available and equally effective. For the providers of care, there are no easy solutions: empathy and listening do help, but they may not be enough. Mind you, if you do get it right it makes the job all the more enjoyable.

Finally, as a number of chapters in this book remind us, an illness or disorder in one member of a family affects the others. That is why family doctors are so important and why the relations and reactions between family doctors and families need to be understood. This critical interface of health care delivery is not perhaps as exciting as gene research or molecular biology, but in my view it is just as important to the development of the practice of medicine.

Sally Wyke and Jenny Hewison have produced a book which has a lot to say to anyone involved with the delivery of child health care: purchasers and providers, voluntary and statutory agencies, within and without the Health Service, and specifically for Health Visitors, School Nurses, Family Practitioners and Paediatricians.

David Hull
Professor of Child Health
Nottingham University

Acknowledgements

This book was based upon an original idea by Professor Meg Stacey, who wanted the research on community child health care undertaken under her general direction at the University of Warwick, to reach a wider audience. We are very grateful to Meg for the support and encouragement she gave us in the early stages of planning this collection, although all the errors and omissions are, of course, our own. We would also like to thank Patricia Fisher, Bill Hill, Kate Hunt, Jean Leiper and Lindsay Macaulay for enormous practical help and psychological support in the panic to prepare the final manuscript, and Patricia Fisher and Lindsay Macaulay for their work in preparing the index.

Chapter 1

Introduction

Jenny Hewison and Sally Wyke

Most child health care is carried out by parents. Up to 90 per cent of minor illness episodes are diagnosed and treated at home;[1] it is parents who decide whether further advice and assistance are necessary, and seek out doctors, health visitors, or other health professionals. In the field of developmental surveillance, it has recently been authoritatively acknowledged that 'parents are far more effective than professionals in the early diagnosis of a wide range of handicaps'.[2,3] The rather well-worn phrase 'partnership with parents' begins to acquire real meaning as we recognize and accept parents' status as principal providers of community child health care. In the Britain of the 1990s, the vast majority of child care is still provided by mothers. Although the balance of child care responsibility between women and men might change in the future, the research presented in this book reflects the world as it is now, not how it might be, and certainly not as it should be. Thus when we refer to parents, we infer, for the most part, mothers.

From the point of view of health professionals, the amount of caring which parents do, and the difficulties which they face in making the 'right' health decisions, are not visible in day-to-day practice. Surgery and clinic staff see only the children whose parents decide they need to be seen. In the nature of things, staff do not see the children whose parents decide – rightly or wrongly – that a consultation is not required. Thus community health professionals see only the 'tip of the iceberg' of children's illness dealt with routinely by parents.

Even though both parents and professionals have children's best interests at heart, they often do not agree about the wisdom or desirability of particular courses of action. 'Best interests' can, after all, carry a variety of interpretations. From the professional's point of view, an inappropriate consultation does not help the individual child concerned, and takes up time that could have been spent helping other children; but the same encounter, viewed from the parents' perspective, might have ruled out alarmingly serious diagnostic possibilities, and provided much appreciated general reassurance.

In these and other circumstances, such as failure to attend an antenatal appointment, a gap exists between the needs and characteristics of service users, and the functions and characteristics of a health service as seen by its providers. We believe that it is in everyone's interests to reduce this gap as much as possible – to bridge the information gap. Service users would be more satisfied with the service they received, and providers would be more satisfied with their jobs. It would also, of course, be more efficient of everyone's time and energy if the service were even more appropriate to clients' needs.

The conventional response of practitioners who recognize that patients are not using the services in ways they consider appropriate, is to say that parents need to be educated in how to use the service. Social science observers of the system have retaliated and argued that health professionals need to be educated about the concerns, beliefs and behaviour of their patients. As they point out, the 'service' in health service refers to the needs of *patients*, not those of the *providers* of care. However, the need for professionals always to be prepared to learn from their patients is by no means uniformly accepted, as the following quotation makes plain (the author is writing in the 1980s, about general practitioners):

> *Paternal v. fraternal care . . .*
> Currently, because of the work of many behavioural scientists there is much concern with the autonomy, health beliefs and status of the patient. . . . There are strong countervailing arguments. The doctor may not know what is best for his patient, but he is likely to know better than the patient himself. . . . The patient's health beliefs may be interesting, but mainly because they are misconceptions to be dispelled. The doctor's health beliefs, however partial and incomplete, may be thought to be at least an improvement on folklore and fantasy.[4]

The writer goes on to point out that although he has deliberately over-emphasized the argument, he does believe that 'the freedom of the patient, his rights and the bounds of his autonomy reside in the freedom of choice to enter medical care and to choose one's medical adviser'.[4]

In this book, we take the view that professionals and patients have much to learn from each other. The apocryphal patient in general practice who demands antibiotics to treat a common cold needs to be educated towards more rational behaviour; even if other information makes the patient's concerns understandable, the antibiotic remains inappropriate. The knowledge that an antibiotic is inappropriate is technical knowledge that needs to be shared. But, equally, parents (usually mothers) have intimate knowledge about their child's health, and how they respond to illness and treatment. Being able to share this knowledge with professionals would lead to more sensitive care, appropriate for each individual child.

Doctors and other health professionals are really quite good at standing up for themselves; they also have good opportunities for doing that. Their status is valued both by the wider society and by their patients, and so they bring more power to interactions: they *can* tell a patient that a consultation was not strictly necessary; as service providers, they can and do convey their views to patients and their parents. Patients, however, have less confidence in speaking up, and they can end up undermined, disgruntled and no wiser.

Patients' needs are very difficult for the individual health professional to identify. For example, one general practitioner may have 2000–3000 patients; their views will be quite diverse and difficult to summarize; patterns will be difficult to discern, even if the individual service provider had the time and opportunity to take a systematic look – which of course, most do not. This means that heavy users of the service, or users whose behaviour seems to be inappropriate to the provider, come to feature prominently in the mind. In these circumstances, stereotypes readily form, and may then acquire self-reinforcing properties of their own. For example, the young mother of several children who seems to come to the health centre with every cough and cold, yet does not turn up for immunizations, may be stereotyped as 'over-anxious, but disorganized Mum'; every consultation could reinforce this image.

The systematic data-gathering exercise that would be necessary to obtain an *accurate* picture would, of course, be prohibitively expensive; while mass-action initiated by patients to convey their collective views to health providers is very rare in this country, and tends to be confined to large and controversial issues.

The National Health Service (NHS) is being led down an increasingly consumerist road. In the view of the NHS put forward in the White Paper *Working for Patients*,[5] it is envisaged that patients will convey their views via the marketplace. It is assumed that patients will 'shop around' until they find the kind of service that they want. The rhetorical aims of the proposed changes are to ensure responsiveness to consumer needs; however, the effectiveness of such a system in reaching its aims has not by any means been demonstrated. In other respects, the proposed new arrangements may actually weaken the consumer voice; for example, since they do not fit in with the marketplace model on which the plans are based, Community Health Councils have no clear role in the current plans. Past and current services are not responsive to consumers, and this was one of the main failings that the NHS reforms were designed to remedy; but the new consumers envisaged in *Working for Patients* are even more passive creatures than the old, receiving information but not giving it, and certainly not being involved in planning the services they need.

Why 'child health matters'?

The justification for this book is based on a simple premise: health care providers and planners need as much information as they can get about the users of their services. This remains true if the motive is altruistic (concern that patients should get a good service appropriate to their needs), pragmatic (efficient use should be made of health professionals' time), or indeed financial (market forces ensuring that services will prosper if they respond to consumer demands). Research has a role to play in providing information. Good research can provide an objective, if not always impartial, view of the world; a view which providers – by virtue of their active involvement in that world – find almost impossible to obtain for themselves.

This volume has been put together to make more widely available information relevant to the planning and provision of health services – specifically, child health services, at community and primary care levels. This information has previously had a more limited circulation, perhaps through publication in learned journals, or in papers presented at academic conferences.

It is important to stress that the information contained in this book was not necessarily collected specifically with service implications in mind. Still less was it collected with a view to writing prescriptions for changes in the working practices of particular types of health worker. The editors of this volume are professional researchers, and it is not their intention – for they would not presume – to teach practitioners their trade. Rather, the spirit and justification of the book is to offer information. This information was collected for a variety of purposes; but all of it is relevant to, and has implications for, the planning and delivery of health services in the context of the British NHS. Research is expensive, and its results should be used. Often this means justifying change; but in the present-day NHS, where change has come to be an article of faith, it may also be used to justify keeping things that work well as they are.

The information in the book is offered at a time when British society is changing very fast. As we have said, most child health care is provided by and within families; but the family of the 1990s is undergoing a major transformation. The proportion of families who are of overseas origin has changed substantially: in 1971, 2.5 per cent of the population of England and Wales were born in the New Commonwealth countries and Pakistan. By 1987, the figure had doubled. In 1971, 47 per cent of married women were in employment; this figure rose to 60 per cent by 1987. Patterns of child-rearing, especially those influenced by material resources such as access to toys and space to play, are very different from those documented by the Newsons in 1963 and 1968.[6,7]

The provision of health services has acknowledged, if not yet adequately responded to, the implications of some of these changes. Hospitals, for example, try to cater for the dietary needs of people from different religious and ethnic groups. By contrast, the provision of an interpreter service is woefully inadequate, despite the visible need for such a service. Other changes in society, such as the increased participation of women in the labour force, seem to have been acknowledged grudgingly, if at all; and the unfortunate impression has sometimes been created that health practitioners are attempting, in the manner of King Canute, to order back the tide.

Another theme must be introduced here. In many specialist domains, such as the antimicrobial properties of drugs, the opinions of health professionals can be acccepted as superior – in the sense of better informed – to those of their patients. The fact that this is true in some domains does not, however, make it true in all; many topics relating in particular to the care and upbringing of children remain 'a matter of opinion'. Indeed, much of current medical practice and advice about infant feeding or developmental play has not been shown to be effective according to rigorous scientific criteria. This is not to assert that information and knowledge acquired through scientific research is the only valid kind. Of course, knowledge acquired on the job or through experience is valid and valuable knowledge, but parents also have a great deal of experience, so disputes about what is 'right' can seldom be resolved on that basis. In the end, it is only training that distinguishes health professionals from their patients, and the expertise derived from that training which justifies the belief that professionals 'know best'.

Professionals and clients in the context of health care

Compared to a health delivery system in which providers have a business relationship with their customers, a system based on the provider as professional has much to commend it. Medical knowledge and clinical autonomy are here sacrosanct, and used to further the client's best interests. The drawback is that the unequal distribution of knowledge that char-acterizes the professional/patient relationship can lead to inflexibility, and an assumption that, by definition, the professional *always* knows best, even on topics which do not form part of his or her legitimate area of expertise.

A health delivery system based on this relationship runs the risk of becoming unresponsive to the needs of its users, and indeed of appearing to promote the interests of professionals above those of their clients. The British NHS has been deservedly criticized on these grounds, and a move towards a more 'user-friendly' service would receive widespread public support.

As we have stated, the Government claims that legislation currently before Parliament will achieve this goal. The plan is to change the nature of the relationships between the three main interest groups in the NHS: pro-fessionals, patients and third parties (particularly managers and Govern-ment). Although there has been much rhetoric about how the changes will make the NHS more responsive to the needs of consumers, the actual legislation is almost entirely about the relationship between professionals and managers (and through them, with Government). More specifically, it is about curbing the power of professionals, by increasing the control that managers can exert over them. In this model, consumers 'have their say' principally by *choosing* from the different services that the new-styled NHS will make available to them; so organizational arrangements designed to incorporate consumer interests into the *planning* of services cease to be really necessary.

The role of information

We said earlier that the purpose of this book is to offer information. The offer was certainly not formulated with a market model of the NHS in mind, but the irony is not lost on us that, in a different context, at least part of what we are doing could be construed as a kind of market research. Organizations that have always operated in the marketplace recognize the value of 'knowing the customer'; the launch of a new confectionery bar is preceded by months, if not years, of analysing who eats what and why. A NHS that was *truly* user-friendly, whether inspired by the political right or left, would want to know more about its users, and to learn from them how its services could be made better and more appropriate to their needs. We hope that the information collected in this book, based on research carried out throughout the 1980s, will help all professionals to 'know their customer' and understand their perspective.

The organization of the book

The rest of the book is divided into four sections. Section 1 contains a chapter by Jennie Popay on the subject of money and having enough of it. Most of child health care is, as we have claimed, provided by parents, who bring resources of expertise, beliefs and values to the task. It would, however, be fundamentally misleading to convey the impression that no other kinds of resources were involved; this chapter reminds us that choices are heavily constrained when financial resources are inadequate. When asked what sorts of things women need to be 'good mothers', rich and poor women alike stressed the importance of personal qualities. 'All you need is love' was a recurring theme; and financial factors were said to be of little significance, even though lack of money in fact placed severe restrictions on the ability of some of the women to care for their children. The denial was understandable, because for many of the women, acceptance would have amounted to an admission that they themselves were not 'good mothers'.

Section 2 contains three chapters. The first two look at interactions with health services in general from the point of view of mothers; the third examines the different perspectives that mothers and health visitors bring to the subject of caring for children, and shows how such differences can have a negative effect on the interaction between them. The chapter by Sarah Cunningham-Burley and Una Maclean asks how mothers recognize symptoms of illness in their children; they argue that health and illness are morally laden categories, and that the decisions that women make are used to judge how good they are as mothers.

The authors found that mothers' recognition of symptoms drew heavily upon their direct experience of children and, in particular, what their own child was 'normally' like. Although most of the time they had confidence in their ability to make health decisions, interactions with health professionals could threaten this confidence, and make them feel that their competence was being put to the test. Thus rather than supporting mothers in caring for their children, interactions with professionals can sometimes undermine them.

Professionals who share the same cultural and language background as their patients may have difficulty enough putting themselves into the patient's shoes. Problems multiply when language is a barrier, and cultural differences are pronounced. This may mean that very little is actually offered by the health service to mothers from certain minority communities, such as the Pathans who are the focus of Caroline Currer's chapter.

Pathan mothers felt that children 'were their business'. As did the mothers in the study reported in the previous chapter, they felt confident in their ability to bring up children, and rejected claims to expertise that were based on less first-hand knowledge than their own. As the author points out, 'an unmarried white health worker might . . . command little respect as an advisor concerning child care'.

Like mothers everywhere, the Pathan women had many competing demands on their time. Also like mothers everywhere, they were helped in setting their priorities by values stemming from their religion, their sense of duty to their family, and so on. Potential difficulties arose because the culturally specific ideas held by Pathan mothers were not necessarily the same as the culturally specific ideas held by white health workers and brought with them to their jobs.

Finally in this section, Berry Mayall's chapter returns to the theme of the source of the knowledge held by mothers and health professionals. The health visitors in her study tended to draw mainly on book knowledge in the views they expressed, and regarded that knowledge as factual. This went along with a view of child care that emphasized the numerous tasks and duties that mothers had to perform in guiding their children through the different developmental stages. Mothers, on the other hand, drew on practical experience as the source of their expertise, and saw their children as people in their own right from a very early age. In the author's words, 'parents did not see their children as tasks'. The theme of resources for care also recurs in this chapter. For many of the mothers, paid work was the only way they could maintain an adequate standard of living for their family; doing such work was intrinsic to good child-rearing as far as they were concerned. Health visitors put much more emphasis on the psychological work of mothering, and felt that in all but exceptionally needy cases, mothers should be full-time carers of their children.

The chapters in Section 3 take a closer look at how parents use health services on behalf of their children. The first two look specifically at general practitioner services, while the last looks at the use made of a variety of services in an inner-city area.

The material in the chapter by Sally Wyke and colleagues is drawn from a study of general practice consultations for children's coughs. Having established that children from materially deprived backgrounds were more likely to be taken to the doctor with their coughs, the author asked if this was because their parents 'overused' the general practitioner service, as has sometimes been claimed, or because the children were in fact suffering from more serious illnesses.

The usual problem in doing research in this area is that information about the seriousness or severity of the illness episode is only available for children who *did* consult, and no comparison is therefore possible with episodes for which parents judged a consultation was not necessary. This study was unusual in that it had access to a severity measure designed to be administered by a non-medically trained interviewer, which collected the same information that a practitioner could obtain during routine history taking.

When consulters and non-consulters were compared across a range of social backgrounds, it was found that the relatively high consultation rates seen in the more materially deprived families could be explained by the greater severity of the illnesses that their children suffered from. In other words, the study did not find evidence that this group of parents was overusing the general practitioner service, but rather that their children's need for the service was greater.

The study reported in the next chapter by Andy Clarke and Jenny Hewison looked at general practitioner consultations in practices serving multi-ethnic areas. Sikh and Muslim parents seemed to consult the general practitioners more often than did white or Afro-Caribbean parents for their children's respiratory illnesses; but once again, the severity of the illness episode did seem to be the chief factor in whether or not a parent would decide to consult. Health beliefs may have contributed to some extent; in all ethnic groups, for example, parents who were pessimistic about the prognosis of an untreated cold were more likely to consult. A greater proportion of Asian parents tended to hold such pessimistic views, possibly stemming from their experiences in the Indian sub-continent, where cold-like symptoms may be indicators of a more serious illness such as tuberculosis.

Two recently published studies have confirmed increased general practice consultation rates in families of Asian origin,[8,9] one of which[9] has suggested that for Pakistani families, the increase might be confined to boys. Neither of these reports contained information from parents on their reasons for consulting, so further research is needed to clarify the issues involved. Both reports did conclude that the ethnic composition of inner cities was likely to influence the workload and case mix of general practitioners working in those areas. Because workload and remuneration for doctors are likely to become increasingly strongly linked, the issue is certain to appear more frequently on the agendas of medical politicians. That being so, the need for more research designed to *explain*, not just document, increased consultation rates among certain minority groups becomes ever more pressing, if the right kind of service is to be provided in the future.

Elizabeth Watson's chapter reinforces the point that parents do not consult without a reason. The London-dwelling Bengali mothers in her study did make greater use of health services than their indigenous counterparts, but they also lived in very much more disadvantaged physical circumstances, and reported worse illnesses in their children. The non-English-speaking mothers in this study were prepared to travel miles to see a Bengali-speaking doctor. They also greatly appreciated the interpreter provided at the child health clinic. Such a facility was notably absent in the antenatal clinics attended by the Pathan mothers in Caroline Currer's study; and at the risk of stating the obvious, the standard form of provision is indeed to provide nothing at all.

The last section of the book differs from the others in that it is not organized around a single theme. Chapters 9, 10 and 11 are on topics that most health professionals will encounter in their everyday practice; Chapter 12 is about HIV infection and AIDS, conditions which are still thankfully beyond the direct professional experience of most people, but which will inevitably be more commonly encountered in the future.

Robert Drewett's chapter reviews research data on a number of aspects of breastfeeding that might prove helpful as guides to future practice. This is again a topic with considerable moral overtones. Strong claims continue to be made about the psychological as well as the physiological benefits of breastfeeding, and women who do not adopt this method of feeding are sometimes made to feel both guilty and inadequate. This would be regrettable enough if the benefits were indeed well substantiated; in fact, there is no sound evidence at all for some of the postulated psychological benefits of breastfeeding, either for child or mother.

There do seem to be real gains to the physical health of the child from breastfeeding, but even these have been well established only in non-industrialized countries where not all families have access to a clean water supply and adequate sanitary conditions. The first study to provide unequivocal evidence of a beneficial effect of breastfeeding on childhood infections in Britain was published in 1990.

Heather Fletcher's chapter is about asthma. This is a more common condition than is often appreciated, affecting perhaps 10–15 per cent of children. Drug developments have revolutionized its treatment in recent years, but there is still a great deal of under-treatment, and up-to-date methods need to be much more widely applied. As with many other chronic conditions, most of the ongoing care of a child with asthma is done by the parents. New knowledge needs to be shared with them, because the best way of managing asthma is to ensure that everybody involved understands the nature of the condition and what to do about its symptoms.

The subject of Jenny Kitzinger's chapter is child sexual abuse. When a child has been abused, the mother's role is vital in helping the child survive and overcome the effects of the abuse; however, this chapter reminds us that mothers have needs too, which should not be forgotten. Mothers of abused children are often faced with an overwhelming sense of guilt and failure, which contacts with health professionals can sometimes serve to reinforce: the mother can be made to feel responsible for 'allowing' the abuse to happen. This allocation of blame influences the way in which help is offered to the mothers of sexually abused children; their needs are seldom met, and the central role that they play in ensuring their child's recovery is often overlooked.

Children who have been abused may suffer from psychological problems that are difficult for their mothers to cope with, and mothers can be left depressed and psychologically exhausted. At such a time, a mother needs all the help and support she can get, but she may feel ambivalence about seeking support from professionals, because the same people whose job it is to provide support are also responsible for surveillance of the family. Admitting one's difficulties might in these circumstances feel like admitting one was inadequate as a mother after all.

Some of the issues that emerged in the context of child abuse are also applicable to the care of children with HIV or AIDS. Children with major problems are being cared for by mothers whose own needs for care are very great; it therefore makes no sense to discuss child health care without also considering the health needs – physical or psychological – of their mothers.

Most children with HIV contracted it from their mothers. Jacqueline Mok draws on her experience in a paediatric counselling and screening clinic in Edinburgh to review community care needs of children with HIV. Most mothers of children with HIV are either injecting drug misusers, or partners of injecting drug misusers. Providing child health care often meant not only dealing with serious, perhaps even terminal, illness in a young child, but doing so in the context of an ill parent and all the problems of multiple social and material deprivation. The author points to the need for a co-ordinated approach, and specifically for shared care between health and social services. She states: 'the lack of a definitive cure for HIV infection does not imply that nothing can be done to help HIV-affected families'.

Most cities and towns in the UK have so far been spared the need to develop a comprehensive service for children with HIV or AIDS. In the event that they are called upon to do so, the lessons learned in Edinburgh may provide a useful guide through this new and hitherto almost uncharted territory.

References

1 Spencer, N. J. (1984). Parents' recognition of the ill child. In MacFarlane, J. (ed.), *Progress in Child Health*, Vol. I. London, Churchill Livingstone.
2 Polnay, L. (1989). Child health surveillance: New report highlights value of parental observation. *British Medical Journal*, **299**, 1351–2.
3 Hall, D. M. D. (ed.) (1989). *Health for All Children*. The Report of the Joint Working Party on Child Health Surveillance. Oxford, Oxford University Press.

4 Marinker, M. (1986). Performance review and professional values. In Pendleton, D., Schofield, T. and Marinker, M. (eds), *In Pursuit of Quality: Approaches to Performance Review in General Practice*. London, Royal College of General Practitioners.
5 Department of Health (1989). *Working for Patients*. London, HMSO.
6 Newson, J. and Newson, E. (1963). *Infant Care in an Urban Community*. London, Allen and Unwin.
7 Newson, J. and Newson, E. (1968). *Four Years Old in an Urban Community*. London, Allen and Unwin.
8 Gillham, S. J., Jarman, B., White, P. and Law, R. (1989). Ethnic differences in consultation rates in urban general practice. *British Medical Journal*, 299, 9553–7.
9 Balarajan, R., Yeun, P. and Soni Raleigh, V. (1989). Ethnic differences in general practitioner consultations. *British Medical Journal*, 299, 958–60.

Section 1

Resources for care

Chapter 2

Women, child care and money

Jennie Popay

Every training course for health professionals includes material on poverty and deprivation. Students are told that for some people caring for their own and their children's health is made more difficult by the poverty they experience. Often, however, students are faced with a morass of indigestible data and with complex multifaceted explanations for the link between poverty and ill-health. Obviously, poor housing, a poor diet, a lack of safe play space, etc., will have a direct effect on children's health. But what is also obvious is that standards of 'parental' care may vary within different income groups. The poor may also be more likely to indulge in health-damaging behaviour, notably smoking, and they may spend their limited resources in ways considered inappropriate. Health professionals sometimes claim to be left paralysed with indecision in the face of such complexity. So much so, perhaps, that they lose sight of the fact that poverty is at least partly to do with not having enough money. One aim of this chapter is to restate this simple truth. But it seeks to do so in a somewhat unusual way.

First, no 'hard' factual data are presented. Rather, the chapter is concerned to present women's accounts of the importance of money to good child care in their own words. Secondly, it does not only look at the experience of poor women, but includes accounts from women living in households at very different income levels – from the very rich to the very poor. In this way it is hoped to provide a sharper definition of what it means for women as mothers to be poor. The intention is to shift the focus away from what poor women *do* and how they *behave* as mothers, to what they cannot do, simply because they do not have the money to do it. This perspective should encourage health professionals to question the somewhat dominant tendency today to view poverty as a cultural rather than an economic phenomenon.

The second aim of the chapter is somewhat different. It is to set discussions about poverty within a broader context than that provided by the traditional focus on low-income households. By considering the experience of the affluent, it is possible to illustrate how women may experience 'relative poverty' even in high-income households, because they lack control over resources. This perspective should alert health professionals to the possibility that poverty can exist in apparently comfortable middle- and upper-class households, as well as in areas of 'multiple deprivation' and among those on low incomes.

The chapter, then, has a dual purpose: to stress that poverty is in large part about the shortage of money rather than about how it is spent, and to suggest that it is also about lack of control where money may not be short. The chapter is therefore concerned both to contrast the experiences of mothers caring for children on widely different incomes and to highlight the similarities in the lives of these mothers.

The chapter is divided into three main sections: the first is concerned with the things that women perceive to be important to them in order to be 'good' mothers and with how money fits into these accounts; the second considers what aspects of child care money can and does buy and compares women's experiences in households with different levels of income; and the final section explores the way in which lack of control over money unites women across different income levels.

The study and the women

The six women whose accounts are provided in this chapter, all took part in a study of patterns of health and health care among parents, based at the Thomas Coram Research Unit at the Institute of Education in London during 1985–8. The study included a series of interviews over a year with men and women in 18 London households. The women are drawn from six of these households. Their names and some details of their lives have been changed to ensure confidentiality. As the cameos below suggest, they lived in vastly contrasting situations, though their own perceptions of their standards of living do not always reflect these stark contrasts.

Liz Pound is a 23-year-old lone parent living on supplementary benefit (SB)[1] with small earnings from a job in a pub. She lives in a small council flat with her 3-year-old daughter Laura. Her total income, after rent is paid direct, is £40 from SB and between £10–30 from the pub, i.e. between £59–70 per week. She has no savings. She describes herself as 'fairly poor I suppose'.

Audrey Tress is a 33-year-old married woman living with her unemployed husband and two children, Paul aged 14 and Teresa aged 11. They live in a three-bedroom council flat on SB of £90 per fortnight after rent and fuel is paid direct, and earnings of around £20–25 a week from a cleaning job, i.e.

around £65–70 a week. She notes that they 'don't have enough money to cover all the basics – it's not enough'.

Anita Brett is a 38-year-old married woman living with her husband and two children, Nick aged 14 and Tricia aged 11, in a council house. Her husband brings home around £600 per month and Anita brings home £250 a month from a part-time job, i.e. a total household of around £850 a month after tax. She describes the family as 'not exactly destitute, like unemployed people, but not well off, somewhere in the middle I suppose'.

Mary Taylor is a 38-year-old woman living with her husband and two children, Mark aged 6 and Sara aged 4, in a semi-detached, owner-occupied house in the suburbs. Mary works full-time earning around £30 000 a year, while her husband looks after the children full-time. They also own a cottage in the country. Mary describes them as 'very much upper income to someone in the lower range, but we wouldn't be considered rich – between middle and upper'.

Emily Corder is a 44-year-old married woman living with her husband and two daughters, Ann aged 18 and Pat aged 15, in a large detached house in a village outside London. Emily has been a full-time housewife since Ann was born. Her husband earns £60 000 plus a year and has many occupational benefits. Emily described the family as 'very comfortable, in the top 10 per cent of incomes'.

Julia Preston is a 31-year-old married woman living with her second husband and two children from a previous marriage, Simon aged 5 and Tina aged 7. Julia is a full-time housewife and mother with a full-time live-in nanny. Her husband earns in excess of £70 000 a year and also enjoys considerable occupational benefits. They live in a large terraced house in central London. Julia notes that 'we must be upper income'.

'All you need is love': resources for mothering

When asked directly what sorts of things they think women need to be good mothers and how they would rank them, these women more or less consistently stressed the importance of personal qualities, such as love, patience and an ability to listen, or factors such as time and a loving family environment. There was a clear tendency among the poorer women to suggest that money was not particularly important.

Audrey Tress, for example, living on SB with her unemployed husband, argued that though they had little money, they had the things that were important for caring for children:

> We might not be rich in money, but we're rich in love and that's what counts. . . . I'm not saying that if I had money there wouldn't be a lot of things that I would buy because there is . . . but we're rich in our own way. I'm not saying that material things don't matter at all, but they're not that important.

Indeed, there was a sense in which money might actually be a bad thing. As Liz Pound, the lone parent argued:

> I think that you learn from not having, you appreciate the value of money . . . in a way I'd rather struggle to get things and have the satisfaction of getting them like, than have it on a plate.

Certainly, it was suggested that people might want more than they 'needed', a sentiment expressed by Anita Brett in the low-paid family: 'You obviously need the money to give them the things that you want to give them . . . but you always want more than you've got don't you?'

The more affluent women also tended to downgrade the importance of money. Julia Preston, for example, the richest among these six women, living on a household income well in excess of £70 000 a year, noted that the important thing was to do the best one could for one's children, whatever one's income. Similarly, Emily Corder, living in a household with more than £60 000 a year, noted that:

> It all depends on what sort of character you are, if you're satisfied with basic needs, you don't need much money . . . as long as you've got reasonable housing and your family's reasonably fed.

As other writers have shown, there are heavy moral and social pressures on women as mothers. They are expected above all to be loving and caring, qualities that are generally seen to transcend the material necessities.[2,3] It is perhaps not surprising, therefore, that women themselves would argue that financial resources are of little significance to the successful enactment of their role as mothers. For poor women to suggest that money is important to their ability to be a good mother would be tantamount to admitting that they could not be good mothers because they did not have money. For all women, it would be to denigrate the personal qualities and skills that give the role meaning and value to them.[4,5]

These descriptions of the importance of different types of 'resources' to 'good mothering' can be termed public accounts.[6] These women tended to relegate money to a minor role because it would be socially difficult for them to acknowledge anything different. However, in their descriptions of their experiences as mothers more generally, they provided a somewhat different evaluation of the importance of money. Here, they painted a picture in which access to money is central and in doing so they highlight the profound disadvantage experienced by women who are attempting to care for their children on very low incomes.

Poverty and plenty: differential access to money among women

For Liz Pound and Audrey Tress living on SB, the absolute shortage of money structured their lives and generated considerable anxiety. Both described an existence dominated by trying to make ends meet and frequently failing. In the face of electricity debts, for example, Liz had switched off all electrical appliances and arranged for a card meter to be installed so that she could pay off the debt. She bought food on a daily basis as she was not using the fridge. She had large catalogue debts. This was partly for clothes, a carpet square and bits of furniture for her flat. However, her purchases were modest and they had no table to eat off. It was also partly because a friend had been unable to pay her bills. Liz's account of how she managed demonstrates that, as well as having more direct effects on living standards, poverty can squeeze out time for caring. Describing her life in general she said:

> It's like I get my money on the Monday and by the Thursday that food will be gone and I've got to wait until Saturday (when I get paid at the pub) to be able to go and get more. So I do manage like that . . . but it's just food and bills and the worrying about covering it. . . . Sometimes I realise that it's days since I've given Laura a hug, which is awful, but things just get on top of me.

For Anita Brett, living with her husband and two children on a low income from employment of £850 a month, things appeared to be somewhat easier. But it is evident from her account that the household budget was tightly balanced and could easily be upset by a large unexpected item of expenditure. As she noted: 'There have been times when we've been a bit short of money or something . . . and you do wonder what you're going to do about it.'

Despite their very low incomes these women would go to great lengths to try to provide extras that they felt to be important for their children's welfare and development. Liz, for example, had struggled for two terms to find the money to send Laura to playgroup because she felt it was important for her. However, she had only recently stopped because she had been using the food money to pay the £25 half-term fee. Anita similarly budgeted carefully to ensure that her daughter could attend a gymnastic class four nights a week, a commitment that also involved a considerable amount of Anita's time taking her to the gym and her husband's time bringing her home. Anita and her husband were also trying to save £500 for Nick to go on a school trip abroad. Plans to put away £50 a month has not worked well, but they were going to be able to get the money from the husband's Christmas bonus.

These women's accounts also show how extended family members or friends are an important source of financial and other support for many families. Liz Pound's parents, for example, had bought her a washing machine, paid for her travel to their home outside London and bought many things for Laura. Anita Brett had not been on a holiday for some years, but this year they were going to a holiday camp with an older couple who were friends of longstanding and who were paying for the holiday. Audrey Tress and her family, who were experiencing long-term unemployment, had no close kin networks, but frequently mentioned reciprocal arrangements with one particularly close woman friend. All three of these women living on low incomes noted at some point that they would like more money, but their ambitions were far from extreme. When asked what she would do if she had more money, for example, Audrey commented that:

> If there was something, like a new carpet or something, I could just go out and buy it and also a holiday, it would be nice to just go abroad for two weeks.

Similarly, Liz noted:

> I'd like better housing conditions, a dishwasher, less financial worries . . . it would be nice not to have to worry about when the gas bill comes in and things like that and family holidays would be nice.

Access to money also featured prominently in the lives of the three more affluent women, but in qualitatively different ways. The management of money did not dominate their daily routine as it did the poor women. However, access to considerable financial resources was a prerequisite for the things they felt to be important in their children's lives. Paramount among these was education. In all three high-income households, the parents had decided to 'invest' in a private education.

These mothers also stressed the value of other activities, such as swimming, dancing, music, gym and riding, that their children were involved in after school and that had to be paid for. Additionally, money provided for a whole range of extra labour-saving devices, from dishwashers to second cars.

It was not the case that money was considered to be limitless in these households. Indeed, in two of them, the private school fees and other activities were described as involving a strain on the family budget, but it was considered to be money well spent. In talking about her children's education, for example, Mary noted that:

> Money gives us the opportunity of hopefully creating a healthy environment for our children. We're fortunate to be in a position to choose to send our kids to private schools, but we do choose to spend our money that way.

Similarly, Emily commented on the pressure on her husband:

> He's earning a living to keep his children . . . it must be a tremendous pressure on him, he must always be thinking of school fees, the horses, etc., and I'm dependent on him . . . there are times when I feel that I am stretching him financially.

In the most affluent household, Julia too was conscious of the importance of money to her as a mother. Not only did it pay for private education and a wide range of extra-curriculum activities, it paid for a live-in nanny, regular holidays, etc. As she succinctly puts it: 'I'm not saying that money is the answer, but it sure can help.' Indeed, in a revealing comment, Julia noted that being a mother came easily to her, but with the proviso that:

> I have always had people to help, so it makes a hell of a difference. I

think I would be quite good at it funnily enough, if I had to do it from the word go . . . but whether I would be good at it from the point of view of all the practical things and I'm not sure I would be very good at it from the point of view of playing with little ones for hours on end . . . I don't need to amuse these ones. I can take them with me to something that amuses me . . . but as I say it came easily because I had help.

In describing their daily lives as mothers, these women are therefore providing what might be termed 'private' rather than 'public' accounts of motherhood. When they are asked to talk about what they do, rather than to talk about motherhood in more abstract terms, they are perhaps less constrained by the 'need' to meet what they perceive to be the social expectations attached to motherhood. In these accounts, it becomes clear that money does make the domestic work go around smoothly. For more affluent women it ensures that they are able to obtain the services that *most* mothers consider to be important for their children's proper welfare and development with relative ease. Additionally, it buys them time and peace of mind, commodities that can make it easier to love and care for children.

The restricted lives of Liz, Audrey and Anita, dictated by a lack of money, and exacerbated by their desire to do their best for their children, is therefore thrown into sharp relief.

Given these contrasts, it is perhaps difficult to imagine that there could be similarities in the experiences of money among the six women, but there are. These similarities arise in relation to the control that women have over the financial resources available in the household.

Whose money is it anyway? poverty amidst plenty

Other researchers have described the different systems of money manage-ment that exist within households.[7,8] Among these six households, two of them – Audrey and her unemployed husband living on SB and Anita living on around £850 a month from her own and her partner's paid jobs – ran a 'whole wage system'. That is, all of the money coming into the household went to the women. Their partners then received pocket money from the women for their own use. The women were therefore responsible for trying to stretch the limited income to cover all communal outgoings. However, none of this money was seen to be available for women's private consumption. Audrey, for example, described how her husband received pocket money of £20 out of the £90 fortnightly SB cheque, from which rent and fuel had already been paid direct. She had the rest of the money, but knowingly comments:

But I don't have the freedom with it . . . by the time we've done the shopping, paid the insurance and the Provident, we buy Joe's tobacco, Joe buys some of his and I buy some, there isn't really a lot left . . . if I needed something I could go and get it, but sort of say: 'well, that tenner's for me', the answer's no. It's gone, the money just sort of diappears so fast.

Similarly, Anita described how she managed all the money because if her husband did it they wouldn't have any! Out of the household income of £850 a month, which went into a joint account, he got £160 spending money. This included travel to work. Anita gets money out for shopping and if she wanted something else she says she would draw out more or sign a cheque. But as she noted, 'The children usually come first . . . I rarely spend money on myself.' Indeed, in seeking to save for her son's holiday abroad, she had stopped travelling to work on the train and went by bus. This took much longer, but she explained it was cheaper.

At the top end of the income scale the household systems of money management differed. Emily, with two teenage daughters, received a monthly allowance of £750 to cover food for the family, some other items of household expenditure and various animals, including the horses. She also had a credit card. The major items of expenditure, including paying the credit card, were organized and paid for by her husband, whom she described as 'more methodical' than herself.

Julia described their system as 'chaotic'. She had her own bank account, which her husband transferred money into 'when the overdraft becomes too large'. Julia estimated that she spent around £1000 a month on household outgoings. The payment of many household items was done on an *ad hoc* basis by either partner, although the mortgage and one of the two cars was paid for through the husband's work. Julia also had a 'nest egg' which she had inherited. A complication in this household's finances was that the two children were hers from a previous marriage and all their expenses – school fees, food, clothing, nanny, a car – were covered by an allowance from their father.

Despite the level of housekeeping monies available and the potential to obtain money from other members of the extended family, or credit, etc., both of these women expressed discontent at the lack of their own money. Julia, for example, talking about how she would like to get a job, noted that:

I don't just want to earn money for money's sake, but it would be nice if one was earning a bit, because apart from anything else . . . it's nice to feel you are paying for your own whatever, rather than always getting money from somebody else or using your own nest egg. I'd use it on the things it annoys me having to spend somebody else's money on, my clothes, presents to other people, you know, all the totally unimportant things really.

Similarly, Emily explained how she had taken a part-time job at one time because she felt she wanted money of her own. However, this had caused problems and more recently, therefore, she had had another idea:

I got very depressed because I was thinking of how it drains him and I would like to contribute and I've always found it difficult, as I was financially independent before I married, to rely on a husband. He's always said: 'No, you're doing a good job, that's why I'm here, to pay for you to do this.' I've accepted it for a bit and then times come when I think I feel useless and then I went out and got this job and I found I couldn't get his supper and the children were suffering. So the other day I thought, 'Well okay, he says I'm doing a job of work. I want to be independent', so I went to him and I said: 'Look, I can't go out to work because of XYZ', and I just explained that, 'I think I'm worth at least £50 a week, so I will take a slight cut in housekeeping and have two accounts – one you will pay £200 a month, which is like my wages and the other will be housekeeping and continue as normal.' 'No problem', he said, 'You're right'. So, from my point of view I feel much better, I don't feel guilty that I have to go and say please or crawl, crawl, crawl.

This system was instituted during the study and she explained at a later interview that she felt it was working well.

Across these income groups, therefore, in two-parent households with the women not earning from employment, they shared a sense of their own lack of access to money that they could consider to be their own and which they felt free to spend on themselves. The more affluent women were less likely than the lower-income women to do without things for themselves. However, in order to obtain resources they had to experience a degree of humiliation: as Emily commented, 'crawl, crawl, crawl' to their partners. Where they did have control over their own money, it also tended to be spent on other people. Anita's nest egg, for example, was to be used to pay for the school fees of future children. Emily was spending some of her newly acquired 'wages' on the children and on decorating a room.

It is in this sense that women share a common experience of relative poverty even among plenty; relative, that is, to others in the household. In this context, it is interesting to note that older children may enjoy equal, if not better, access to money of their own, than their mothers. Two children in these households had monthly allowances of around £60 to cover what were described as 'minor expenses', and one had a car of her own bought by her grandparents.

What then of the other two women? Liz Pound, the lone parent, and Mary Taylor in full-time paid employment. Liz clearly had control over all the resources coming into the household. Indeed, she had described how her ex-partner had squandered money from the social security benefit on clothes and entertainment, while she struggled to keep the household afloat. This had eventually led to arguments, to severe violence and then separation. However, despite now having control, she felt ambivalent about her right to money from the state:

I don't feel right taking it. I mean I have to because I have no choice. . . . I just don't feel right about it, you know. Like people think: 'Oh, another single parent getting everything free', and it isn't nice to be like that. But there are circumstances when you've got no choice. I mean I tried to work but it didn't pay.

This attitude, at least in part, probably influenced her decision not to claim some of the extra monies that she was entitled to and to insist on attempting to pay in full for her daughter's pre-school care, despite the fact that she could probably have obtained a subsidized rate. While Liz was therefore not in a subordinate position to a male partner, she clearly felt that the power and control lay with the state. Her experience of the money she received was shaped by social values which she felt labelled her as undeserving.

Mary, in contrast to all the other women, had control over her own money. Indeed, her situation powerfully illustrates how the disadvantaged position of women is created by the sexual division of labour between the domestic and the public sphere rather than because they are women *per se*. Mary is a successful businesswoman and she and her partner had decided that he would stay at home and look after the children while she remained in the formal labour market, as she could earn more. For Mary this was not a problem:

It's my money . . . not that I see it like that, it's family money. I would certainly not buy anything major without consulting him, but I certainly wouldn't consult him on a pair of shoes for me, or clothes.

In contrast, her partner explained that the worst thing about being at home with the kids was:

Not having my own money. It's her income, though we do have a joint account, it all goes into the joint account, but I don't really spend any, well it's not really my money.

This man suggested that this attitude might be 'Just a mental hang-up of mine . . . a very male attitude . . . not having one's own money.' However, as the women's accounts suggest, it is in fact likely to be a feeling common to all of those – overwhelmingly women – who provide unpaid domestic labour and who do not have paid employment.

Conclusion

It is apparent from these women's accounts that there are enormous differences in women's access to money across social classes. Additionally, whatever their public accounts, the lack of access to money among some women does place severe restrictions on their opportunities to care for themselves and their children as they would wish to do – opportunities that are clearly available to the more affluent. Poor women go to great lengths to provide the material things that they feel to be important for their children.

Being a 'good mother', therefore, involves both personal qualities and financial resources, but these may be in conflict. The struggle to meet the social expectations of being loving and caring while living in poverty undoubtedly blights the lives of women and children in ways that are all too apparent when one considers the privileges of the more affluent.

A focus on women's experience of living at very different income levels, therefore, serves to throw the disadvantage experienced by the poor into sharper perspective. However, it also points to those dimensions of inequality that bind women together, regardless of household income. The social structures and ideologies of gender cut across those of social class. They begin in childhood and stretch across the labour market years into old age, tying women firmly into domestic roles. These roles restrict their access to the labour market and therefore their control over financial resources, creating relative poverty within even the richest households.

So what are the implications of all this for people in health and social services working with mothers? First, rather than decrying the ignorance and irresponsibility of the poor, it is important to recognize the wizardry with which they manage meagre resources and the resilience and initiative that helps them to survive on a day-to-day basis. Many health workers already do this. But there are still those who blame the victims of poverty for their plight. It is particularly important that health workers are sensitive to women's pivotal role in managing poverty within low-income households. This may entail considerable stress for women, and insensitive professional interventions may exacerbate this.

Secondly, health workers need to be sensitive to the way in which women's lack of control over money may lead them to neglect their own needs, even in more affluent households. This dimension of women's experiences of poverty points to the importance of ensuring women's access to money in any strategy to promote the health and well-being of mothers and children. Child Benefit, for example, is a vital component of such a strategy, as it is paid directly and universally to the main care-giver – normally the mother. Similarly, access to good quality paid employment is also important, which in turn means the provision of housing and affordable child care for instance.

There are, of course, limits to what individual health and social service workers can do in relation to the dimensions of poverty discussed here. But we are a long way from reaching these. Health workers can make much more of a contribution than they do at present to extending women's rights and their access to resources. Welfare rights work with those on low incomes is the most obvious aspect of this. But health and social service workers could also attempt to gain a working knowledge of a range of locally based initiatives that might be relevant to women's needs, including, for example, employment training agencies.[9,10] More generally, there is an important role for professionals to act as advocates for those they serve. What Clement Attlee argued[11] some 70 years ago for social workers should equally well be applied to all those in the health and social services:

> The social worker must have definitive views and must have formed some clear conception of what society he [sic] wishes to see produced. . . . I think it is a mistake for him to hold aloof from social

reform movements. . . . The social worker has as much right to make clear his views as anybody else. . . . Every social worker is almost certain to be also an agitator. If he or she learns social facts and believes they are due to certain causes which are beyond the power of an individual to remove, it is impossible to rest contented with the limited amount of good that can be done by following old methods.

Acknowledgements

The research on which this paper is based was undertaken as part of the ESRC-funded programme of research within the Centre for Studies in Education and Family Health, an ESRC Designated Research Centre at the Thomas Coram Research Unit. I am grateful to the parents who agreed to take part in the research and to Charlie Owen who has helped me with the use of software for the qualitative analysis of text.

References

1 The interviews took place before Income Support and Family Credit replaced Supplementary Benefit and Family Income Supplement.
2 Finch, J. and Groves, D. (eds) (1983). *A Labour of Love: Women, Work and Caring*. London, Routledge and Kegan Paul.
3 Graham, H. (1983). Caring: A labour of love. In Finch, J. and Groves, D. (eds), *A Labour of Love: Women, Work and Caring*. London, Routledge and Kegan Paul.
4 Oakley, A. (1974). *The Sociology of Housework*. London, Martin Robinson.
5 Boulton, M. G. (1983). *On Being a Mother*. London, Tavistock.
6 Cornwell, J. (1984). *Hard Earned Lives: Accounts of Health and Illness from East London*. London, Tavistock.
7 Pahl, J. (1980). Patterns of money management within marriage. *Journal of Social Policy*, 9(3), 313–35.
8 Brannen, J. and Wilson, G. (eds) (1987). *Give and Take in Families*. London, Allen and Unwin.
9 For a more detailed discussion of this issue, see Popay J., Dhooge Y. and Shipman, C. (1986). *Unemployment and Health: What Role for Health and Social Services?* London, HEC.
10 Dhooge, Y. and Davis, M. (1989). *Working with Unemployment: A Training Manual for Health Promotion*. South Bank Polytechnic, London.
11 Attlee, C. (1920). *The Social Worker*. London, Bell.

Perspectives on health

Chapter 3

Dealing with children's illness: mothers' dilemmas

Sarah Cunningham-Burley and Una Maclean

Most health care takes place in the community, indeed within the private confines of the home, and most providers of such health care are women.[1,2] Child health care is no exception.[3,4] It is mothers, primarily, who attend to their children's health needs: who make daily decisions regarding their well-being; recognize the early stages of their illnesses; and nurse them when sick. This they do amidst other commitments, for other relatives, partners, for domestic and paid labour, and alongside their overall responsibility to provide an adequate, indeed, healthy environment in which their children will grow and develop, with whatever resources are available to them (see Chapter 2, this volume).

As a society, we expect an enormous task of our mothers, and off-load an onerous responsibility on to them. In the study presented in this chapter, we wanted to find out about how mothers dealt with the daily grind of health and illness in their young children: How did they recognize illness? How did they decide what to do? How did they feel about their contact with health care professionals? It is only by knowing more about what is going on in the community, that child health services can reflect and respond to needs, for the better promotion of child health generally.

Investigating the cultural context of children's illness

To develop an understanding of how mothers deal with health and illness in their children, a method of investigation has to be used that places emphasis on mothers' points of view. The study we conducted was exploratory; we wanted to find out as much as possible about mothers' perceptions of health and illness, and their decision-making behaviour. We did not want to predefine what was meant by health and illness, or appropriate action, as these were taken to be culturally defined concepts and actions.

We used unstructured interviews, based around a topic guide that was developed from pilot work. We aimed to cover a range of issues that might be relevant to understanding the cultural context of children's illnesses, yet also to encourage the mothers participating in the study to talk about what was important and relevant to them. Such qualitative methods have been found to be particularly appropriate to understanding women's experiences,[5,6] and provide a non-threatening environment that encourages the development of rapport between the researcher and researched.

This last point is particularly important in a study of this kind. As Backett[7] has noted, '. . . just as respondents may find it personally threatening to have a researcher question their taken-for-granted modes of family behaviour, so also current emphasis on personal responsibility for health makes it a far from neutral topic for investigation'. We had to ensure that the mothers felt relaxed and confident that their point of view was being taken seriously, and that they were not being judged.

We found, on the whole, that the mothers interviewed talked willingly and well about their children's illnesses, many saying that they enjoyed having the opportunity to do so. However, we also identified a tendency to assume that our interest must be in the more serious illnesses, rather than with the everyday ups and downs of children's health, which were considered hardly worth mentioning. Thus, it was memorable episodes that sprang to mind when the mothers were asked to talk about their children's health:

R54: I cannae remember to tell you the truth — the ear infection has always stuck in my mind.

Routine illness had to be made an important topic in its own right. This meant going beyond the public account,[8] which tended to stress the healthy aspects of their children:

R58: I have been very lucky with both of them as regards their health. If you looked up the medical records you would see there is very few entries from them . . . they get coughs and colds, but they are very healthy.

The women had to be encouraged to talk about the boring and mundane, to make important all the hidden health work that they do.[9] In-depth methods were the only ones that could achieve this.

Additionally, we utilized a healthy diary, so that we could collect information on a day-to-day basis. Again, this was unstructured, and provided useful information that complemented the interview material. The diaries recorded what the mothers did daily to monitor and attend to their children's health and well-being.

A total of 54 women, with at least one child under the age of 5, were interviewed. All but one were married, and the median age was 28 years. A further six women were interviewed for the pilot study. All but two of the women contacted agreed to participate in the study. The interviews were all conducted by S. Cunningham-Burley, lasted between 40 minutes and 2 hours, and were tape-recorded and transcribed. A total of 42 health diaries were completed, totalling 927 days when information was collected. The study was carried out between 1983 and 1985, in a new town in Scotland.

Preliminary health care work

As we have noted above, most health care takes place outside the professional arena; it is mothers who are at the front line of primary health care. They monitor closely their children's well-being.[10-12] It will usually be they who first recognize that their child is or may be ill. As has been reported elsewhere, our study found that the mothers were alert to small changes in behaviour that might suggest that a child is sickening for something,[13,14] as well as noticing physical symptoms such as 'runny noses'.

It is mothers who know what their child is normally like. In addition to being responsible for a child's health and nursing that child when sick, a mother is involved in all types of care and activity. Health and illness are embedded in everyday life, and are not dealt with as separate issues:

> **R62:** They haven't had any sort of illnesses or things like that. They both coped with going to playschool quite easily, and she went away to school quite happily and she settled down alright.

Because mothers know what their children are normally like, it is not surprising that we found that they could quickly identify deviations from normality. These deviations were related to notions of health and illness, and were often causes of some concern.[9] What is of particular interest is the mothers' own assessment of this process. They were aware of their unique abilities, although they could not necessarily give a precise account of what they did, as the following example demonstrates through the use of the word 'sense':

> **R68:** I think it helps if you are with her all the time. You know what to look for. That's my opinion anyway. I feel you can sense when she's going to be ill.

The mothers, then, were well aware of their skills, and had considerable confidence in their ability to recognize that 'something was wrong' with their child or children:

> **R35:** It's a funny thing with mothers – you can tell when they're no well.

Their unique ability is borne from accumulated experience of their own child, and his or her normal self. They develop a unique stock of knowledge, through which they interpret changes in a particular child:

SC-B: What sort of things do you normally look out for then if you think they are sickening for something?

R17: Well, in the case of these two if they do start to cry a bit more than normal. . . . Both of them are not cry babies unless it's really something.

Each child is different, and mothers respond to this. Thus, although you have more experience generally with subsequent children, you still have to develop knowledge specific to each child:

R50: . . . you get signs, and all the kids are different. If *she* is not really well, she stops eating.

R56: He's a lot easier to recognise it. He's totally different. She . . . from food wise, she picks at her food anyway, but he'll sit and eat it, and if he doesn't want his meals it's because there is something wrong with him and he is very quiet and sort of sits and cuddles in, whereas he is usually away playing and quite happy by his self. She's different, it's not until she's white as a ghost or too warm or that, you say, oh there's something wrong with her.

Notions of normality, which underpin the mothers' recognition of illness,[9] extend beyond knowledge relating to an individual child. Normality is a cultural product, and the mothers drew on commonsense knowledge, and culturally approved knowledge to make sense of their children's health and illness. This knowledge derives from peers, professionals, parents, the media and 'what we all know about children and mothering'.

Beliefs about normality, then, shape definitions of health and illness. Normality is related to different developmental phases: behaviours may be treated as normal at certain stages but not at others. A baby not eating would be treated as a worrying deviation; a toddler not eating may be having a 'fad'.

A concern for health in a general sense underpins the mothers' ideas of normality, and reactions to deviations from the normal. A normal child – one who develops well, eats and sleeps well – is healthy. Such a child may get ill, but some minor illness in children is seen as normal and not treated as a threat to health:

R25: But as I say, we've never had much experience of anything. They've never had anything to really worry about other than normal childhood illnesses.

Therefore, a healthy child may suffer from normal childhood complaints, such as colds. Yet, changes in behaviour which are considered an essential part of normal, healthy development often gave cause for concern;[9,14] they may threaten healthy development, or portend illness. Eating and sleeping concerns were particularly important for the mothers, and were mentioned in all the interviews as the mothers talked about health, illness and their worries.

Changes in behaviour were not simply interpreted as clues to some underlying problem; their relationship to illness was more complex. In fact, whether or not illness was present was not necessarily the primary concern for the mother. A mother may be concerned generally that her child is not eating or sleeping enough, and may therefore not develop healthily. Changes in behaviour may be noticed before the onset of an illness episode: indeed, an illness may not even materialize. The diaries demonstrated such monitoring with the subsequent 'back to normal'. As we have noted elsewhere,[15] changes in behaviour could be treated as precursors to illness, the result of illness, the problem itself, or a problem for the family in general.

Health care and maternal competence

It is not surprising that behaviours associated with normal, healthy development were considered to be important by the mothers in our study. Society emphasizes the nurturing role of the mother and her role in ensuring the adequate physical and emotional development of her children. Health and illness are thus morally laden categories and, as Prout has pointed out, 'Child health care is a central component in the definition of proper motherhood and it is one of the axes around which judgements of maternal competence are made.'[16,17] Decisions that mothers make regarding health and illness can thus be treated as measures of 'appropriate mothering'. Some of what the mothers told us in the interviews show that they were acutely aware of these pressures; and, more subtly, that concern to deal appropriately with the children's health and illness was tied with concern to be *seen* to be dealing appropriately. Appropriate mothering becomes a moral imperative, underlying mothers' reactions to their children's illnesses. No one has to actually say anything to them for the mothers to feel that their competence is being questioned, by health professionals, or by others in general:

R17: I used to get bothered that he would lose a lot of weight and they would think I'm no feeding him.

R52: I suppose you want your baby to look nice all the time. You're no wanting folk to look in the pram and think oh my God my bairn's sick . . . things like that used to worry me.

As we noted above, changes in eating and sleeping behaviours were important concerns for the mothers. Many said that they were worried that their child was not getting enough to eat:

R40: I think this is what was wrong with the bairn, you know. He wasnae getting enough to eat sort of thing, he greet [cried] all the time.

And not-eating may be a reason for seeking professional advice:

R68: If Nicole was really ill, like if she was off her food and that, I

> would go to the doctor . . . but the way I feel, as long as she is eating and that, and she is running about quite happy, so there's nothing to worry about.

In some situations, it may be the 'not-eating' rather than the illness that is the mother's worry, and health professionals need to recognize and respond to these different relevances. The mothers' descriptions of their children's sleeping problems created a vivid portrayal of the difficulties which they had in coping with a wakeful child, not always knowing what was wrong, and not getting enough sleep themselves. Nursing a wakeful child could cause problems for the whole family, and professional advice to leave a child to cry was considered difficult to follow:

> SC-B: And did you find that quite a problem for the first few years?
> R48:   It is because like the doctors and the nurses, and the health visitors say: 'Just put her down and shut the door, and let her cry.' But it was hard, I mean we tried it for a solid hour and you've got a tiny baby crying for a solid hour, it's hard just not to go in and see her.

As Graham has noted, a mother may experience acute feelings of responsibility and inadequacy as her baby cries.[18] Concern with eating and sleeping behaviour provides part of the cultural setting within which health and illness are managed. They highlight issues of adequacy in the mothers. A bad mother is one who does not look after her child adequately, and this can be represented through a child who cries a lot, or does not take his or her food properly. A mother's self-esteem is intricately bound to her child's behaviour and development.

Interaction with health services

It is no wonder, then, that the mothers' interactions with health care professionals were sometimes marked by ambivalence and dissatisfaction. Once the mother decides to seek outside help over a problem (and it should be noted that this was the least likely response to minor illnesses),[13] her competence is much more open to scrutiny, and thus her self-esteem under threat. The mothers' confidence, evident in how they spoke about recognizing something was wrong in the first place, did not extend to interactions outside the mother–child dyad. There is much more brought to the interaction than the immediate concern for the child's health.

Feeling stupid

The mothers did not make the decision to consult lightly. In fact, out of 456 days where the mothers noted in their health diaries regarding their children, only 20 resulted in a general practice consultation; 2 in home visits, and 2 in phone calls to the health centre. Yet, it was common for the mothers to describe themselves as feeling stupid or silly in regard to their contact with general practitioners. They did not use the same vocabulary to describe contact with pharmacists, who were often used by mothers as part of their repertoire of responses to illness in their children.[19,20] While some expressed dissatisfaction with the health visiting service, again they did not use the same vocabularly to describe how they felt. It seemed to be the doctor–patient relationship, in particular, which could result in a mother saying she 'felt stupid'. This has to be understood in the context within which women mother, and deal with health and illness. As we have said, their self-esteem may be under threat if their child's health, or their management of the child's health, is open to scrutiny and their 'mothering' is being judged, however implicitly. General practitioners may be quite unaware of this context and, importantly, the doctor need not use phrases implying that the mother was stupid, or reacting inappropriately. The mothers sometimes felt this anyway:

> **R59:** You felt silly if you phoned the doctor and he said just bath her down. I had to do that many a time, all night, just to keep her temperature down.

Here, the advice itself seemed to make the mother feel silly, rather than providing her with the reassurance that she could competently deal with the situation herself.

> **R58:** I remember we called Dr. Z in one day. Joseph must have been about three and he came out in these wee spots all over and of course there had been measles, and everything on the go and I thought he's got measles, and it was an allergy. I felt so stupid.

Making distinctions between serious and trivial illness is difficult for both mothers and doctors, and the mothers sometimes found it difficult if they had consulted over something that turned out to be nothing much to worry about. This could make them feel stupid as the above example illustrates. As Howell has noted: 'mothers are variously blamed when their children become ill: for bothering the doctor too often, for not having brought the child in early enough, for being unduly alarmed, for not having recognised signs and symptoms of "real" illness'.[21] The mothers may not actually be blamed, but they were vulnerable to feelings of being stupid or silly, which could easily be reinforced if their concerns were not dealt with sensitively:

> **R12:** . . . and he [the GP] says 'Oh no we don't want to bother with that' . . . and it really made me feel 'Oh you stupid woman', you know. He says 'You mothers, you worry yourselves sick over silly little rashes. I'll give you another cream . . . and that will work.'

A vocabulary of neuroticism was available, and used by the women to express how they felt they were sometimes seen. Again, this has to be understood within the wider context of the position of mothers in our society:

> **R15:** I think the doctors thought I was neurotic. He [child] had a cough and I kept on thinking there was something wrong with him and the doctor kept on saying he would grow out of it. It was a terrible cough and everytime I went along I am sure he said 'Oh not her again'. . . . I am sure I could see it on the man's face.

A fear of being seen as over-reacting, or being over-anxious was often evident in the mothers' descriptions of their decision making and interactions with doctors. Yet, at the same time, they are burdened with having to make decisions about their children's illnesses, and not to let a serious condition develop.

Not bothering the doctor

The mothers' accounts of their views on their doctors, and on whether they should consult, were also dominated by the theme of not wanting to bother the doctor and of not wasting his time. This provides further understanding of the wider cultural context within which mothers make their decisions. Again, this is tied to the problem of distinguishing trivial from serious problems, and to the different relevances of doctors and mothers. Some were concerned that they might be consulting inappropriately, thus 'bothering the doctor':

> **R62:** Sometimes you think, well is it worth bothering him, but so far, what they've had, if it hasn't cleared up within a couple of days I sort of try to make an appointment to see the doctor or call him in. . . . I know there must be people that 'phone up just for anything and they've got to be sure that you need a doctor.

Mothers' behaviours could sometimes be curtailed by this concern, so strong is the imperative that one should not waste the doctor's time:

> **R47:** I got to a stage that I wouldn't go to him because I felt like he was . . . here she comes again just purely wasting his time . . .

Again, the general practitioners themselves may not have intentionally given any indication that they thought their time had been wasted, but this shows how important it is to consider the way the mothers might be interpreting what is going on, and what concerns and vulnerabilities they bring to the interaction.

Doctors were considered to be busy people, with many demands on their time. While there was some feeling that there should be no question-marks surrounding whether to attend to a young child whom the mother was concerned about, many other events would seem less clear-cut. Even on occasions when the mother herself felt in no doubt about the appropriateness of her demand, the doctor is still portrayed as 'busy':

R11: He might have been held up. I don't know. He apologized when he saw what she was like anyway, but it wouldn't have helped if she had died. But I suppose they are run off their feet and you cannae expect anything else.

The mothers' views on their interactions with general practitioners may be grounded in both a general sense of what they thought doctors do, feel and say, and perhaps a personal experience or particular episode where the mother felt she had been made to feel that she had consulted inappropriately.

Being responded to as competent carers

The mothers talked about what they wanted or expected of their general practitioner. It was clear that they wanted to be treated and responded to as competent, not neurotic or overreacting women. For them, this would mean that their concerns were treated seriously, even if the illness was self-limiting and could be treated by care at home. They felt that the general practitioner should spend time explaining what, if anything, was wrong. They certainly did not want just to get a prescription, and were prepared to learn from advice well-given:

R28: Because a few times when they've had a cold, Dr Y's said to me 'what have you done?' Well, given the junior . . . or half a . . . and that sort of thing. Well, I mean you're doing everything that's possible and that's that. I'd rather be said that than sort of said nothing and given you a bottle and you don't know what the bottle is for. I would prefer that the doctor would say 'You're doing everything you can. I can't help you anymore', but at least you are settled in your mind and you've been and there is nothing else so you just come back and get on with it.

Reassurance was often an important element in the interaction; either reassurance that nothing else more serious was going on, or that the mother was responding appropriately with whatever she was doing at home:

R5: Dr W will say, 'I don't think she needs a bottle. Just you keep giving her . . .'. Well, I'd rather have that, whereas before any other doctor I went to, they'd gie you a bottle to shut you up, ken.

Deciding to consult a general practitioner does not mean the mother is expecting a cure or a prescription; it may be an important step in deciding whether the child is really ill, or an opportunity to learn whether she is doing the right thing, or whether an alternative treatment could be recommended. It is after all the mother who has to go home to nurse the child giving cause for concern, and the consultation should make that activity as appropriate and as easy as possible, with advice and reassurance.

Implications for child health care

Child health care services in the community must be grounded in a good understanding of what mothers do, day in day out, for their children. Health care professionals need to be aware of 'the central and essential contributions made by mothers to promote, maintain, restore and protect the health of the children'.[21]

One way of doing this is to recognize that the mothers usually deal with children's illnesses without recourse to professional help or advice.[13] When they do contact health services, it is often after considerable deliberation. There are strong norms militating against consulting unnecessarily: the women did not want to bother busy doctors, nor to be seen as neurotic or overacting.

In a consultation, effort should be made to show the mothers that their ability to recognize something wrong is treated seriously, and that their concerns are considered important. Mothers' concerns with soft non-specific symptoms and signs are different from those of health professionals. The nature of mothers' concerns must be recognized – is she consulting because she is worried that the child is not eating, or because the child may be ill with a medically defined condition? Is she worried because the child does not seem to be improving although home care has been provided? The exact reason for consulting a professional at this point in time should be elicited. The professional should make certain that he or she does nothing that might reinforce mothers' feelings of vulnerability, and should aim to boost mothers' confidences in their health care activities. Opportunities for health education should be taken up and executed sensitively. Mothers should be considered as an integral part of the primary health care team, and a fundamental element of community child health care.

References

1 Stacey, M. (1988). *The Sociology of Health and Healing*. London, Unwin Hyman.
2 Ungerson, C. (1983). Why do women care? In Finch, J. and Groves, D. (eds), *A Labour of Love*. London, Routledge and Kegan Paul.
3 Mayall, B. (1986). *Keeping Children Healthy*. London, Allen and Unwin.
4 Davis, A. (1982). *Children in Clinics*. London, Unwin Hyman.
5 Oakley, A. (1981). Interviewing women: A contradiction in terms. In Roberts, H. (ed.), *Doing Feminist Research*. London, Routledge and Kegan Paul.
6 Graham, H. (1984). Surveying through stories. In Bell, C. and Roberts, H. (eds), *Social Researching, Politics, Problems, Practice*. London, Routledge and Kegan Paul.
7 Backett, K. (1990). Studying health in families: A qualitative approach. In Cunningham-Burley, S. and McKeganey, N. (eds), *Readings in Medical Sociology*. London, Routledge.
8 Cornwell, J. (1984). *Hard Earned Lives: Accounts of Health and Illness from East London*. London, Tavistock.

9 Cunningham-Burley, S. (1990). Mothers' beliefs about and perceptions of their children's illnesses. In Cunningham-Burley, S. and McKeganey, N. (eds), *Readings in Medical Sociology*. London, Routledge.

10 Blaxter, M. and Paterson, E. (1982). *Mothers and Daughters: A Three Generational Study of Health Attitudes and Behaviour*. London, Routledge.

11 Spencer, N. J. (1984). Parents' recognition of the ill child. In McFarlane, J. (ed.), *Progress in Child Health*. London, Churchill Livingstone/Longman.

12 Locker, D. (1981). *Symptoms and Illness: The Cognitive Organisation of Disorder*. London, Tavistock.

13 Cunningham-Burley, S. and Irvine, S. (1987). And what have you done so far? An examination of lay treatment of children's symptoms. *British Medical Journal*, 295, 700–702.

14 Cunningham-Burley, S. and Maclean, U. (1987). Recognising and responding to mothers' dilemmas. *Maternal and Child Health*, August, 248–56.

15 Irvine, S. and Cunningham-Burley, S. (n.d.). Doctors talking to mothers: Concepts of normality, behavioural change and illness in their children. Unpublished manuscript.

16 Prout, A. (1986). Wet children and 'little actresses': Going sick in primary school. *Sociology of Health and Illness*, 8(2), 118.

17 Graham, H. (1984). *Women, Health and the Family*. Brighton, Wheatsheaf.

18 Graham, H. (1982). Perceptions of parenthood. *Health Education Journal*, 49(4), 120.

19 Cunningham-Burley, S. and Maclean, U. (1987). The role of the chemist in primary health care for children with minor complaints. *Social Science and Medicine*, 24, 371–7.

20 Cunningham-Burley, S. and Maclean, U. (1988). Pharmacists and primary care: Some research findings and recommendations. *Family Practice*, 5(2), 122–5.

21 Howell, M. C. (1978). Paediatricians and mothers. In Ehrenreich, J. (ed.), *The Cultural Crisis of Modern Medicine*. New York, Monthly Review Press.

Chapter 4

Understanding the mother's viewpoint: the case of Pathan women in Britain

Caroline Currer

Razia Bibi had been in England for 3 years when I met her in 1980. She had six children, the oldest of which was 20 years old, married and living in Pakistan; the youngest were twin girls who had been born in Britain and were by this time 2 years old. The twins and their two older sisters, 10 and 6 years of age, lived with Razia, her husband and an uncle and aunt and their two children. Razia had told me that she had only one son living with her grandmother in their village in Pakistan. She herself was lonely in Britain, missing life in her village, despite the company of her own sister. She was also physically exhausted caring for her two very lively twin daughters. These girls suffered from 'fits' during which they did not breathe, changed colour and lost consciousness. This would occur if they were upset or reprimanded. Although herself unable to communicate with her GP, these symptoms were reported to him by her husband. The doctor did not recommend any medicine or pursue the matter, merely advising the mother, again through her husband, not to upset the children. She felt obliged, therefore, to give in to all their demands, including a demand to be constantly carried. As they were becoming heavy, this was increasingly exhausting for her. She had had headaches two or three times a week, for which she took painkillers obtained from the chemist, and 'dizzy spells', sometimes daily, which lasted a few minutes and would leave her feeling very weak. She was not too concerned about the twins' 'fits' because their older sisters had been the same in Pakistan. She had taken them to a *malwi* (Muslim priest) who had made a *tarwiz* (prayer amulet) which had helped. The older women in the village and the *malwi* had said that the trouble would last for 7 years and then clear up. This had proved correct, and so she was now confident that the twins' disorder would follow the same pattern. Her own health was a source of more concern – it was not easy trying not to upset 2-year-old twins, especially when they could not run outside as her other children had used to do in the village setting.

How is the health worker meeting Razia to make sense of Razia's own complaints and of her apparent complacency in face of her children's symptoms? He or she is unlikely to have a picture even as detailed as that presented here; in fact, there were in the area in which Razia lived no health workers able to communicate with her directly. In more general terms, it is of course seldom, if ever, the case that health workers have a full picture of the rationale of patients' behaviour in consulting (or not consulting) them, or complying with their advice. In the practical situation, when difficulties of communication and differences of culture are a feature of the health care interaction, the worker's task of understanding the behaviour of patients or their parents becomes even more difficult. While actions may be credited with a rationality, this rationality is inaccessible to the worker and often seen as based upon superstition. Whether more or less tolerantly viewed than a white counterpart, the patient from a minority ethnic group receives no better treatment. Accusations of racism in health care[1,2] may appear to confuse or worsen the position for the practitioner. Paradoxically, it is often the workers trying hardest to understand cultural differences who are the target of such criticism; texts (see, e.g. Henley[3]) which have been found helpful may themselves be seen as racist in the assumptions they embody or promote. Why is this? Can the concerns of theory and practice be brought together? Is there a way forward for those practitioners who are concerned to offer non-racist and sensitive services to all groups?

This chapter addresses these issues. In common with other chapters in this volume, it demonstrates the rationality underlying mothers' decisions in respect of issues of child development and child health care – in this case, the mothers are Pathans currently living in the North of England who have moved from their homeland in the North-West Frontier Province of Pakistan. Most of the children concerned were born in Britain, although many of the mothers had children previously who were born and raised in Pakistan.

Putting the women's own point of view indicates the thought and care that goes into decisions that might, without such an account, appear bizarre, irrational or irresponsible. This presents an inevitable challenge to those too ready to dismiss the mother's experience or expertise. I found women eager to improve the care of their children and to accept help in this, where their own competence and concern was respected and built upon rather than dismissed or threatened. They were quick to know those workers who had confidence in them, despite the difficulties of language, and equally adept at circumventing the aims of those workers who were hostile. The accounts also challenge a number of the assumptions upon which health care is based. Social and cultural assumptions are usually invisible because they are taken for granted; cross-cultural work draws our attention to them in the same way that historical comparisons remind us of changing fashions in child-rearing norms. Social and cultural assumptions have serious consequences when they serve as measures of 'normality' in the area of child development.

Such challenges may appear to make the practical business of providing sensitive child health care seem more, rather than less, difficult. In one sense, this is so, and there can be no doubt that it is an uncomfortable process for those of us in positions of power (whether based on gender, skin colour or professional status) to attempt sincerely to incorporate into our approach the position and views of those to whom we offer a service. Nevertheless, it need not be a process without guidelines. In presenting my research findings, I had to try to discern an underlying pattern or framework in terms of which to organize and understand what the women were telling me about their understandings and actions. Through a discussion of the particular situation and views of the women I interviewed, I shall therefore offer a more general framework which may serve as a useful tool in the attempt to understand the actions of other groups as well as of these Pathan mothers whose accounts gave rise to it.

The research

Razia was one of 17 women whom I interviewed in depth in the course of this project. A further 26 women were also involved and commented to varying degrees. All were Pathans and had moved within the previous 10 years from their homeland in the North-West Frontier Province of Pakistan. All had at least one child under 5 years of age. Their language is Pukhtu and their religion Islam. I had previously worked as a psychiatric social worker in Pakistan among Pathans for 5 years (1972–7); there I had learnt Pukhtu. The research was funded by the DHSS.

Fieldwork took place in 1980–81. During this time, 105 visits were made and 91 interviews conducted, in Pukhtu, by myself and a Pathan research assistant. Like our respondents, we were both mothers: each of us had three children under 5 years of age at that time. Interviews were semi- or un-structured, and focused on five areas: child-bearing (conception, pregnancy and delivery); child-rearing; the woman's own world (social contacts and visiting, dress, religious observance); health and illness (including contacts with health services); and mental well- and ill-being. Although envisaged as individual interviews, they were often in the event group discussions, with a number of women present.

Contact was made, mainly by personal introduction, with Pathans living in five of the major Pathan areas of settlement in the city. Fifty women were contacted, four of whom did not wish to be included in the research. The division of the remainder into 'focus' and 'additional' respondents followed from the women's wish to meet me in a group rather than alone. 'Focus respondents' were those women who fitted my research criteria (Pukhtu speakers with at least one child under 5 years) and with whom I aimed to complete the research schedule.

The respondents

The respondents were all women, all practising Muslims, aged between 19 and 39. Only three of the 17 focus respondents knew their age, but health records and other data gave us reasonable estimates with an average age of 27 years. Only 5 of the 17 had any formal education; of these, 2 were educated beyond primary level. More than these five had learned Arabic in order to read the Koran. All but four of the women spoke very little English; the four exceptions understood more than they were able to use, but did not routinely use the language. However, all but four (a different four) spoke more than one other language fluently – most spoke three languages. None had ever had a job outside the home or expected to do so; all observed purdah, and none went out 'without a reason'.[4] Their length of stay in this country ranged from 1 to 14 years. All of those interviewed lived in the inner-city area and all owned the houses they lived in. Of the 17 focus families, 5 owned a car; 2 shared ownership with close relatives. Seven of the husbands were unemployed; the other 10 were manual workers.

Such details are important as a means of conveying to the reader certain facts about the people whose views are reported. They can, however, be deceptive when a minority group is being considered. Their meaning and implications cannot be assumed to be the same as they might be for other groups. Thus, gender and religion determined many other factors, such as education and employment. In the past, births were not routinely registered in the villages of Pakistan and nor are birthdays routinely celebrated: age has less importance than it has come to assume in Britain. A man's employment following migration may be very different from that which he might obtain in Pakistan, often of lower status. Other factors which might be a source of status, e.g. religious piety or a woman's family background, are not acknowledged or visible to an outsider, although they might continue to be a source of regard within the community.

It is not claimed that those included were representative of even the Pathans currently living in Britain. Nevertheless, their lives and views warrant our attention, both for the general principles that can be discerned and because their situation, although at an extreme, is not an uncommon one. Aspects of their experience are common to women of other groups, including white women, different as their circumstances may appear at first glance.

The issue of play: concepts of child development

The issue of developmental play is one that concerns many child health workers, playgroup leaders and nursery teachers who have contact with Asian families.[2] Mary Whitelock, a health visitor, noted a discrepancy between Asian mothers' views concerning the need to stimulate young children and babies and what she observed as lack of stimulation and attention in the homes she visited.[5] All her respondents thought that having bright toys near a baby would help him or her to move more and to see better, yet none were apparent on visits. Eighty per cent thought that talking to baby would help him or her to talk earlier, yet few seemed to talk to their babies.

There might of course be a discrepancy between stated response and practice, with women either agreeing to an ideal that they perceive to be the 'right answer' for the interviewer or to an ideal that they also hold but cannot attain for reasons of space and/or finance. In respect of this issue, however, my evidence points to a different ideal, both in terms of different goals of personality development and in terms of different processes of socialization.

It is ironic that people in the Indian subcontinent see ours as a culture which devalues and ignores children. In Pakistan, one old man recounted to me in horror that, on a visit to Britain, he had seen a woman carrying a dog and pushing a baby (in a pram). He had remembered this because it seemed to epitomize the strange ordering of values here. In Pakistan, babies are rarely left alone in cots with stimulating coloured mobiles; they are held and passed around. In my interviews, toys were rarely to be seen. Pre-school children were present but did not interrupt. Children were not expected to initiate conversation, but neither were they necessarily excluded from adult company.

Children's behaviour in front of guests was not typical of their behaviour at all other times, as I discovered through staying in the home of my research assistant. There, the upstairs bedroom was full of toys, paper and pens. It was not until I became 'one of the family', however, that the children brought their toys to me. They were certainly cleared away when guests (including researchers and health visitors) called. In all the homes we visited, even the smallest room was kept clean and tidy for guests. Children's toys were not to be seen there. Toys themselves were differently viewed, often seen by parents as rubbish. Mothers were indeed not familiar, it seemed, with notions of developmental play and 'good toys'. I suspect that this was not only for reasons of cost, and that programmes suggesting low-cost options for play (such as wooden spoons and cardboard boxes) would be no help. What women looked for was opportunities such as those they were used to in Pakistan: places outside the home where children could make a noise and run about in safety. Tragically, racist attacks prevented the use of such facilities as were available (see below).

An underlying difference was, however, that child and adult worlds were not separated; the whole 'culture of play' as it has developed here rests on this notion of separate worlds, with their separate equipment – special children's models of household tools such as irons or washing-up bowls offer a good example. In the homes that I visited, young children looked after younger siblings rather than playing with dolls, and helped with household tasks as soon as they were able. I am not suggesting that these children did not want dolls, nor that they did not have them, merely that childhood was viewed differently – indeed, less separated from family life overall – and that the view of toys as an essential part of a child's emotional and intellectual development is a culturally and historically specific one.

This view has come to be a basis for a number of health and educational procedures, assessments and programmes; its apparent objectivity may blind us to alternative patterns, with other bases, which may be as beneficial for the child and may even offer certain advantages – in terms of the development of social skills, for example. To see the children as necessarily unstimulated because they lacked special separate facilities reflects a particular concept of child development, based on notions of individualism that do not fit with Asian family life and are not consistent with many of the values of community which underpin it.

The children's social, as opposed to individual, skills were well developed, but such skills may not be assessed by measures of child development or educational attainment which emphasize individual and intellectual skills. We need to look critically at all such routinely used assessments – poor levels of measured performance may be accurate measures of what they are measuring, but what they are measuring may be a very partial view of the child's overall development. This partiality is racist when we give the impression that children of minority groups are less well developed than white children of their age,[6] or that their mothers are poor raisers of children.

The basis of expertise

Mothers' views of childbearing derived from their own experience. All the respondents had grown up in large families in Pakistan. They had first-hand experience of babies and of child-rearing, albeit in a different context. Inevitably, this experience formed the basis of their expertise as mothers. It was apparent, however, that they were ready to modify their practice on the basis of advice or example when they saw new ways as beneficial or more appropriate in the British context. Many customs were, by virtue of migration, modified for them. Those who had reared children in Pakistan commented ruefully on the comparative ease of mothering in the village: 'I used to let out the children when I let out the chickens.' Life in a small terraced house in the inner city was not easy with seven children. Mothers were actively involved in assessing alternatives where these existed, and in changing their practices accordingly. They were, however, reluctant to modify practices on the basis of what they saw as insufficient evidence presented by health workers. An issue in question is the use of *surma*, a black paste applied around the eyes of babies and young children. Some sorts of *surma* contain lead, and this has given rise to an extensive programme of health education in Britain.[7] Health visitors working with mothers frequently met with resistance to their attempts to dissuade mothers from using *surma*. Mothers' explanations to me were based upon their own knowledge and previous experience. Apart from religious and cultural reasons for its use, they had lived in a place where it is widely used and where any harmful effects were not apparent. They were not convinced by the arguments of women whom they knew had no such experience. They therefore listened politely or pretended not to understand, and ignored the advice given. I am not here questioning that such a danger exists, but the approach taken in concentrating upon this issue, and the unbalanced view that such concentration gives in terms of professional views of Asian mothers' abilities as mothers. The women interviewed considered the health workers' experience less than their own; they also resented the attempt to alter practices that were to them important, without any recognition of the issues involved. The women's intelligence and sense of responsibility formed the basis of their assessments of the advice given, together with a careful and long-term assessment of the personal qualities and degree of understanding of the worker concerned. Their conclusions may have been regrettable in the light of medical evidence, but they were carefully arrived at, and a central issue was their own concern for the health of the child, defined in their own terms.

In matters of infant and child care, the mothers saw themselves as the experts. This is hardly surprising since, as women in a strictly sex-segregated society, children were their 'business'. Moreover, their experience would be extensive, because female children are generally involved in the care of infants in their extended family from an early age. In respect of routine child care, the basis for knowledge and respect was experience, not learning. An unmarried white health worker might therefore command little respect as an adviser concerning child care. However, the women did make a distinction between child care and matters of illness. I asked whose advice they would seek if they had a difficulty with their children, and they replied that they would seek help from an older (more experienced) woman in their community if it was a matter of behaviour or routine care, but from their husband or a doctor if it were a matter of illness. About this they were adamant, having a high regard for the power of biomedicine to heal, although sometimes a poor opinion of particular doctors.

Reasons for difficult choices: interests

I want to turn now to areas of disagreement that highlight the way in which mothers were weighing different interests and conflicting responsibilities. The first is unusual in so far as it is an occasion when women's own personal interests were considered. This is the question of fasting in pregnancy. The Birmingham *Daily News* of 4 June 1987 carried the front page headline 'Babies at risk from Ramadan', in which it reported the concerns of medical experts, as well as the comments of Muslim leaders (men) that pregnant women are not required to keep the fast, provided they make it up by fasting later, but that 'a lot of Muslim women are ignorant about the rules. They don't realise that there is a leeway.'[8] I am not questioning here either the medical concern (although it would be important to see the results of an investigation of this), nor the exemption that exists within Islam. I would, however, question the idea that women are necessarily either ignorant or irresponsible in this matter. All 46 of my respondents were fully aware of both the rules and exemption, and of the concerns of health workers, who tackled them concerning this at antenatal clinic. So what was their own point of view?

Women explained to me that keeping the fast with everyone else was important to them, for a number of reasons. Keeping the full month's fast at the appropriate time was a matter of religious pride and a source of spiritual enrichment. It is also of course much easier to observe the fast when others do, rather than alone at a later time, especially if you are the person responsible for cooking, etc. Because menstruation renders women unclean and so unable to pray, women cannot usually observe the full fast in the normal course of events. Pregnancy may, therefore be the one time when a young woman can keep the full fast. Male religious leaders may fail to realize the significance of this for women to whom religious observance is very important.

Nevertheless, all the women also stated that the health of their baby was of greater importance. They felt able, however, to assess the risk during a particular pregnancy. Health workers advising them not to fast seemed to do so as a 'blanket' condemnation of a practice which they saw as unnecessary. The women, however, were very careful and detailed in their own daily assessments: some with previous difficulties did not fast; others with better past experience who felt themselves to be healthy during this pregnancy did so unless a reason occurred which caused them to stop for fear of the baby's health. They saw health workers as ignorant of the importance to them of their religious observance, as well as underestimating their capacity to act responsibly on the basis of their knowledge of their own health. There are parallels with advice sometimes given that women who are pregnant should necessarily give up work.[9] The women themselves pointed to the evidence of experience, in Pakistan and in Britain, that the practice has not had serious or far-reaching consequences for their ability to bear healthy children, provided that they continue to act carefully and responsibly.

A mother has responsibilities beyond those to one child and to herself as a servant of God, however. There were times when a mother had reluctantly to forfeit the good of one child for the interests of others in the family. As Hilary Graham points out,[10] such conflicts of responsibility are commonplace for all mothers. For these Pathan mothers, keeping antenatal appointments frequently conflicted with the demands of hospitality or the needs of family members. Mothers rarely missed appointments 'for no reason', but they did have to consider their actions in the context of lives where there were many conflicting demands upon them. Because antenatal care was not seen as very important in the context of a concept of pregnancy which views this as a normal condition, clinic appointments might occupy a low place in women's priorities.

Overall, the pattern of reported attendance at antenatal clinic varied, and women's previous experience again influenced their views. One woman stressed the importance of antenatal care on the basis of a previous complication of pregnancy which had been corrected. Most attended, despite considerable practical difficulties (e.g. transport, time off work for their husband, care of older children), because 'it is how things are done here' or because they would receive poorer care during delivery if staff were angry because they had not done so. In view of the difficulties and a perceived lack of benefit in most cases and of the disrespectful way in which they were often treated, it was their continued attendance, rather than any non-attendance, which I found remarkable.

Context of childbearing: options and constraints

I have already referred to the differences experienced by mothers rearing children in Britain as opposed to in the village situation in Pakistan. Constraints were imposed by type of housing, the climate and lack of financial or material resources. Two other important facets of the women's lives further limited these resources: the lack of many members of their own extended family in the migrant situation, and the hostility and racist attitudes they met in the community.

Isolation was not, contrary to expectations, a problem for most of the respondents. It had been supposed, on the basis of various texts[11-14] that women might be isolated, given that they observed purdah and were therefore unable to go out of the home 'without a reason'. In fact, I discovered their patterns of visiting and interaction to be determined by a combination of factors including the availability locally of women from their extended family, the distances involved and the public or private nature of the space to be covered (i.e. whether on open streets or along the house backs). Only 4 of the 17 focus respondents were without anyone who could be visited and could therefore be seen as 'isolated' in the immediate sense. These women all had a strong sense of belonging to family groups, despite the absence of actual contact, but the total absence of casual relationships, such as those that might be formed at the shops or school gate, did mean that this isolation could be quite extreme where it did occur. Other women, the majority, were members of networks in which visiting was frequent, although not always a positive experience for all concerned. These networks did not, however, always offer practical help with child care or housework. While the absence of in-laws led to greater freedom, which was generally valued, especially as women had continually to face the problems of defining appropriate behaviour afresh in the new circumstances of the migrant situation, it did limit the care they received at certain critical times. A good example is that of women returning home following delivery of a new baby.

One of the subjects about which I was asked was infant feeding. All of the women involved expressed a preference for breastfeeding, giving religious, cultural and practical reasons for this preference. Yet only 8 of the 17 focus respondents had breastfed their most recent baby. Of this number, most complained that their milk had dried up prematurely, and they speculated about the reasons for this phenomenon, which all agreed was linked to living in Britain: all had breastfed babies in Pakistan for much longer periods than they found possible here. Again, various reasons were suggested, among which was that nursing mothers here could expect less rest and nourishment than would be provided in the village situation, certainly in the early days following their return from hospital. In Pakistan, other women would prepare special rich food and take care of the housework,[15,16] here, women were on their own, often returning home to unwashed nappies of their older children in addition to the extra work of the new baby. The relatives who would be expected to help were simply not present; neighbours who were fellow villagers would visit to offer congratulations but 'no-one comes to help' (cf Horwitz[17] and Finlayson[18]).

Mothers were further restricted by the lack of play areas and by racist attacks on their children in the streets and local parks – even in their own backyards. Examples given included verbal abuse and physical attacks by dogs as well as other children and youths. Mothers were bewildered by these actions and could not understand how they or their children had provoked them.

Concepts, options and interests

I spoke above of a more general framework that seemed to underlie respondents' reported behaviour. Three areas were identified, those of concepts, options and interests, and I will end by showing how these three categories may help us to discover some of the rationality underlying mothers' actions.

I use the term 'concepts' here to mean the way in which a situation or experience is understood. Such understanding on the part of individuals is clearly a part of and related to more general cultural understandings; it is also related to his or her position in society.[19-21] Thus, Razia's understanding of her children's 'fits', in the example I used at the outset, included the notion that this was a condition that was time-limited and could be helped by prayer. She also understood her own health as of less importance than, and expendable in the service of, her family's well-being. This idea is widely shared, as Pathan proverbs indicate: consider, for example, the saying among women that 'the greater your wealth [of children], the worse your health' or 'though the mother is dry, she must suckle her son'.[22] Ill-health was to be accepted and endured without complaint, the price a mother pays for bearing and rearing children. Women's concept of themselves as mothers was one in which this was their business, in which they were expert. Their concepts and understandings were based on experience rather than learning, and they had a confidence in this experience that perhaps contrasts with the uncertainty of many new mothers. Their concepts of pregnancy were of a normal event that was culturally understated and not discussed in front of men and certain relatives. With an average ideal completed family size of four or five children, pregnancy was indeed both a normal and a routine event for these women.

'Options' is a term I have chosen to use for the practicalities of an individual's situation; the social circumstances such as poverty or wealth that may determine the range of possibilities for action. Razia's options for the care of her twins were fairly limited; by the weather, location and type of house (no garden), and lack of nearby safe play areas. Her options for seeking her own health care were completely limited by the absence of any health worker able to understand her and by her own inability to communicate except in Pukhtu. I have argued that an apparent lack of toys was probably less due to the families' social and financial circumstances than to different concepts or understandings of child development. When we look at antenatal attendance, however, we can see the combined effects of different concepts of pregnancy and of the options, or constraints, upon women, in so far as the appointment would often mean that the husband had to take time off work to accompany his wife for reasons of transport and/or translation. The costs of attendance were therefore high and the benefits not always apparent.

'Interests' have to be considered if we are to explain why two people in similar circumstances and with similar understandings will nevertheless act in different ways. This enables us to include and acknowledge the importance of choice: we are neither the victims of our understandings nor of our circumstances; we decide priorities and, when these conflict, choose between them on the basis of their importance for us. This ongoing process of choice was illustrated clearly in the case of fasting in pregnancy, but it underlies many other situations. Thus, Razia's own ill-health could be expected to become a concern sufficient for her to seek help when it interferes not only with her own life and happiness but with her ability to care for her family. Antenatal appointments might not be kept if a child were ill or a visitor called.

This framework is relevant in understanding the actions and decisions of health workers as well as of their patients. Thus, the health worker's advice or action is determined in part by his or her concepts or understandings of the problem, condition or situation. These understandings have been informed by training but also by personal experience, philosophy and the overall culture. Many tools or procedures used in health care contain implicit cultural understandings that are not open to challenge by individual practitioners because they are invisible. The worker also works within constraints imposed by departmental or government policies, administrative requirements, resources of time or money. These define the options which he or she has in any situation. He or she will then make choices that depend in part on the perception of certain situations as more or less important; more or less amenable to treatment or more or less comfortable or prestigious to deal with.

The framework is one which helps to guard against racism in both research and practice concerning minority ethnic groups. At the risk of oversimplification, it is useful to highlight three common characteristics of racist work. First, there may be a concentration on cultural explanations, to the exclusion of others.[23,24] By this I mean that cultural differences may be seized upon to explain behaviour with less (or no) attention paid to social circumstances (e.g. poverty) which are shared by other ethnic groups. There is also sometimes an assumption that individuals are victims of their culture; without the ability to choose to act contrary to it or to change and modify it by their actions. This was clearly not the case for my informants: I was able to watch as women created their own norms of behaviour in the new situations facing them. This was a complex process in which religious and cultural understandings were of importance, but so too were their own priorities and interests. Thus, while it is necessary to understand and be sensitive to overall cultural patterns and norms, the minority ethnic patient should not be seen as *only* a product of their religion or culture.

Secondly, work may be racist because it fails to examine the cultural underpinnings of health care practice itself; it may implicitly assume that white patients have *no* culture or that health care in Britain is 'culture free'.[23] Biomedicine's claims to universality and objectivity make this a particular danger, and it is therefore possible that neither the *organization* of health care nor the assumptions embodied in biomedicine itself are questioned. Hence my insistence that health workers, no less than their clients, act upon these bases.

A third characteristic of racist work, not included in the framework but compatible with it, concerns the meeting between patient and health worker. There is a danger, perhaps stronger in work that acknowledges the cultural facets of both 'sides' in this interaction, that the meeting will be seen as a meeting on equal terms. It is of course not so.[23] No writing in this area can ignore the realities of unequal power on the basis of races. Black and white do not, in our society, meet on equal terms; nor do health workers and their patients. It becomes the more important that the patient's perspectives are understood and taken account of in the services available and in the way in which they are delivered.

References

1 Brent CHC (1981). *Black People and the Health Service*. London, Brent CHC.
2 Pearson, M. (1986). Racist notions of ethnicity and culture in health education. In Rodmell, S. and Watt, A. (eds), *The Politics of Health Education*. London, Routledge and Kegan Paul.
3 Henley, A. (1980). *Asian Patients in Hospital and at Home*. London, Kings Fund.
4 Currer, C. (1986). Health concepts and illness behaviour: The case of some Pathan mothers in Britain. PhD thesis, Department of Sociology, University of Warwick.
5 Whitelock, M. (1984). An investigation into the expectations Pakistani women in Woking have of the health visitor. Unpublished project report.
6 Griffiths, K. (1983). Child rearing practices in West Indian, Indian and Pakistani communities. *New Community*, **10**(3), 393–409.
7 DHSS (1983). *Surma: Is Your Child at Risk?* London, HMSO.
8 Birmingham *Daily News* (1987). 4 June.
9 Graham, H. and Oakley, A. (1981). Competing ideologies of reproduction:

Medical and maternal perspectives on pregnancy. In Roberts, H. (ed.), *Women, Health and Reproduction*. London, Routledge and Kegan Paul. Also in Currer, C. and Stacey, M. (eds) (1986). *Concepts of Health, Illness and Disease*. Leamington Spa, Berg.

10 Graham, H. (1979). 'Prevention and health: Every mother's business', a comment on child health policies in the seventies. In Harris, C. (ed.), *The Sociology of the Family: New Directions for Britain*. Sociological Review Monograph No. 28. Keele, University of Keele.

11 Saifullah Khan, V. (1974). Pakistani villages in a British city. PhD thesis, University of Bradford.

12 Knight, L. (1978). Protect their minds too. *Mind Out*, 31, 12–14.

13 Wilson, A. (1978). *Finding a Voice*. London, Virago.

14 Schofield, J. (1981). Behind the veil: The mental health of Asian women in Britain. *Health Visitor*, 54, April, May, June.

15 Gideon, H. (1962). A baby is born in the Punjab. *American Anthropologist*, 64, 1220–34.

16 Dobson, S. (1988). Ethnic identity: A basis for case. *Midwife, Health Visitor and Community Nurse*, 24(5).

17 Horwitz, A. (1978). Family, kin and networks in psychiatric help seeking. *Social Science and Medicine*, 12, 297–304.

18 Finlayson, A. (1976). Social networks as coping resources, lay help and consultation patterns used by women in husband's post-infarction career. *Social Science and Medicine*, 10, 97–103.

19 Currer, C. and Stacey, M. (eds) (1986). *Concepts of Health, Illness and Disease*. Leamington Spa, Berg.

20 Ablon, J. (1973). Reactions of Samoan burn patients and their families to severe burns. *Social Science and Medicine*, 7, 167–78. Also in Currer, C. and Stacey, M. (eds) (1986). *Concepts of Health, Illness and Disease*. Leamington Spa, Berg.

21 d'Houtaud, A. and Field, M. (1986). New research on the image of health. In Currer, C. and Stacey, M. (eds), *Concepts of Health, Illness and Disease*. Leamington Spa, Berg.

22 Ahmed, A. (1973) *Mataloona* (Pukhtu proverbs). Peshawar, Pakistan Academy for Rural Development.

23 Pearson, M. (1983). The politics of ethnic minority health studies. *Radical Community Medicine*, 16, Winter.

24 Lawrence, E. (1982). In the abundance of water the fool is thirsty: sociology and black pathology. In Centre for Contemporary Cultural Studies, *The Empire Strikes Back*. London, Hutchinson.

Chapter 5

Ideologies of child care: mothers and health visitors

Berry Mayall

This chapter explores the differing perspectives of two groups of people on childhood and child care – mothers and health visitors. The study focused on the diverse multi-ethnic population for whom the health authority promises child health services. The study has been written up in a variety of papers and a book and these give detailed accounts of the methodology and findings.[1,2] In writing this chapter, I am not attempting to 'prove' anything through a detailed analysis of data. Instead, I point to general features of the contrasting perspectives of mothers and health visitors, consider assumptions underlying their perspectives, and note how these relate to assumptions underpinning models of provision of community child health services – those currently in place and those under discussion.

Background

The mothers

Thirty-three mothers took part in the study, all of whom had a first child aged 21 months. We sampled the women to over-represent ethnic minorities. Fourteen women were born in the UK, eight ethnic majority and six ethnic minority. Of the remaining 19 mothers, 5 had been in the UK for over 15 years, 5 for up to 10 years, and 9 for up to 5 years. Apart from those born in the UK, the other mothers and fathers came from 20 different countries spread around the world. For 14 mothers and 10 fathers, a language other than English was their first language, though in only four cases did we interview parents in another language.

The health visitors

We interviewed a random sample of 28 health visitors, representing all parts of the same health district, and including part-time and full-time workers, specialist and generic workers, fieldwork staff and their seniors.

The interviews

The mothers and health visitors were interviewed three times each, at monthly intervals, using a semi-structured interview schedule. We asked about their views on their daily lives, on child health care, on the health services and on other resources available for parents and children (such as childcare services, housing, transport, local amenities, employment opportunities). The interviews were all tape-recorded and transcribed, and what follows is a summary of their views based on the interview transcripts.

Perspectives on children

Mothers

The women in the study perceived their first, 21-month-old, child as a complete person; as they looked back over the first year and a half of the child's life, they stressed the child's achievement in moving from what she was at birth to 'her being now'. The child was seen as having a clearly defined personality: obstinate, persistent, ingenious, care-free, a worrier, sensitive, cautious, a bully, and so on. Her personality and identity were also revealed in her affectional behaviour. Children of this age actively developed relationships: they initiated cuddles and kisses with people close to them. They were seen as people to interact with, they were company and fun, and they were also trouble when they insisted on getting their own way.

   Mothers saw their children as active in the spheres of learning and social life. The children demanded to extend their knowledge, and they insisted on responses to their questions and to their initiations: they took their parents to coats and outdoor shoes, and opened the door to go out; they insisted on their parents reading with them and playing ball with them. They were keen to take on jobs around the home: they commandeered dust-pans, stirred the cake-mix, did the washing up. They began to take over personal care by insisting on brushing their own teeth, struggling to dress themselves, and taking an interest in controlling excretion, for example. In their social life, beyond that with their parents, they were observed to enjoy interacting with other children and adults, to watch and copy, to play with others and develop relationships with them.

Altogether, three-quarters of the 33 mothers said they found their children more enjoyable now than when they were small, because they were now rewarding, interesting persons. Those mothers who found that being with their children was more difficult now, said their behaviour was difficult – the children were perceived to be frustrated by poor housing and social isolation.

Two points were very noticeable in the mothers' accounts: the child as independent operator and the child as communicator. Looking over the child's life-span so far, mothers emphasized the drive towards autonomy: the child's attempts to take control over certain jobs, to make her own decisions about how time was to be spent. A third of the mothers laid particular stress on the fact, noted with approval, that their children were now much less dependent on parents and were able to play happily on their own or with other children for longer periods without constant reference to parents.

In addition, mothers emphasized that their children had by 21 months become good communicators. For mothers, the acquisition of clearer speech marked a major breakthrough in development. All except two of the mothers referred to their child's increased linguistic competence, when asked how the child had changed recently. From what they said it seems there were at least three reasons why this was an important step. First, the child could now communicate her needs and wishes so was easier to care for. Secondly, there was now more of a two-way relationship: both child and parent could communicate directly through language, so that the child was more fun and better company. Many mothers also described how they could now gain better insight into their child's thinking. Thirdly, language acquisition marked an important socially approved achievement. Mothers have no doubt internalized the messages of the media, the schools and the health care workers, i.e. that speech acquisition both signifies that the child is progressing well and is regarded as critical for a child's success in the educational system.

Health visitors

Health visitors did not see the children at age 21 months so much as persons, but as 'pre-social-objects'. That is, they stressed the socialization process through which a child goes, via a series of developmental stages, towards the goal of becoming a full person. Indeed, they emphasized that mothers' responsibility was to steer children through these stages.

Health visitors put much less stress on the child's part in developing and learning, and far more on the mother's purposeful activity. In their accounts, the child was a relatively passive figure. This vision was evident especially in respect of two topics emphasized by health visitors: control and stimulation.

For health visitors, an important task for mothers was to teach their children to conform to certain social and moral norms: the children should be encouraged to sit down 'with the family' to eat meals; they should have a regular routine, for meals, sleep and daily activities; they should sleep separately from their parents; the mothers should make it clear that they controlled daily life and family norms, i.e. the child must learn 'who's boss'. To all but a small minority of health visitors, it was self-evident that these were desirable norms for mothers to aim for. The question of discipline and how to manage the child was seen by health visitors as a key topic, and especially when the child, from about 18 months onwards, began to develop a will of her own.

Stimulation was a second key topic. A child's learning was seen to depend on the mother stimulating the child. Purposeful stimulation was essential for the child to reach her full potential. Stimulation was important for all branches of the child's learning: the development of motor skills, the development of curiosity about the world, but especially the development of language. The child learned language through conversations purposefully initiated by the mother. This view contrasts very strongly with that of mothers, who found their children initiated learning and learned skills, including language, through exploration and interaction during the ordinary give and take of family life.

Health visitors emphasized their concern that some mothers gave poor child care as regards controlling and stimulating their children. For instance, asked whether their own and some mothers' views about child care differed, all except two thought they did, and thought that these other mothers' ideas were worse than their own. The two topics most commonly referred to were food and socialization. Some mothers gave their children poor food and did not sit them down to regular family meals. As regards socialization, some mothers did not discipline their children properly and many did not stimulate them enough.

Living with children, working for children

Mothers

It follows on from mothers' perspectives on the child as a person, that they thought of their life with their child as life with a new person in the family. That person was small, physically weak, somewhat ignorant and lacking in many skills and so needed care and protection, but these caring behaviours were only one part of life with children. Children were people whom parents lived with, enjoyed the company of, negotiated with, and put up with the faults of, just as one does with older people. Mothers, and fathers, enjoyed teaching their children, but they also enjoyed living with them. It is difficult to put this non-negatively: parents did not see their children as tasks!

Mothers saw their children as members of the family, and of the wider social network. It was important that the child take her place in the social order of the family, as one member of the family, and not always as the centre of attention. This meant that when there was a family event – a visit, a wedding, a funeral – the child took part. If there was an evening party attended by all the relatives, some mothers put a higher value on the child attending than on getting the child off to bed.

The vast majority of mothers saw their children as sociable people, who enjoyed and learned from the company of other children. For a third of mothers, developing relationships with other adults was important too. Childcare provision in nurseries was thus a good in itself for the children, as well as being desirable to free mothers' time and energy.

Finally on this theme, it should be said that while mothers and fathers were interested in the long-term good of the child, they were also interested in promoting the child's immediate happiness and well-being. Thus, while mothers thought sweet-eating was bad for the teeth, children liked sweets and so mothers provided them. Children who seemed happier going to sleep in the company of their parents were often allowed to do so, even if the parents valued the idea of separate sleeping arrangements.

Health visitors

Almost all of the health visitors saw the only important relationship for the child in her first 3 years as with the mother. Within the 'mother–child dyad', the mother should foster emotional bonds with her child, give the child a firm sense of security and stimulate the child to achieve her full potential. It was desirable for the child to develop a relationship with the father, but he had less importance, for the child's capacities were for one principal attachment.

Health visitors saw other social contacts as much less important for the child. Many health visitors perceived it as useful for the child to spend time with other children – if their mothers were there too (as at mother and toddler groups) – because children should learn to be with other children, to share and take their turn. Health visitors saw this experience as standing them in good stead when they reached the age of 3 and began to go to playgroup or nursery school. But before the age of 3, children were perceived as engaging only in parallel play, i.e. copying rather than interacting with each other.

Apart from developing affectional bonds with the child, health visitors saw the most important part of mothers' work as steering the child through the sequence of developmental stages. These were each attended by the likelihood of problems and it was desirable that the mother should know about these in advance so that she might prevent them, or manage them calmly, rather than panic.

So in the health visitors' view, a mother's life with her child included many tasks and duties, which together ideally made a full-time job for her. Making and maintaining a close continuing relationship, controlling and stimulating the child and seeing her through the much charted (but dangerous) waters of child development stages were crucial parts of the package.

Motherhood

Mothers

Most of the mothers perceived themselves as people who also had a child to live with and care for now. The emotions, behaviours and adjustments intrinsic to motherhood were an important part of their identity, but not the whole of it. Most mothers wished to continue with their social lives and with paid work. For them the question so often asked by governments and researchers, 'Why do mothers work or want to work?', was irrelevant. Adult women, whether mothers or not, wish to take part in the normal world of paid work. In our sample, some wished to pursue their careers, others to advance their education, others to take part in the social world of paid work. For many, paid work was the only route to maintaining an adequate standard of living for themselves and their children.

Mothers perceived material goods as important to enable children to live healthy lives. Good food costs much more than poor food. As one mother ruefully said: 'You would think unprocessed food would be cheaper than processed, but it isn't.' They felt children needed spacious safe housing, so that they could run and explore. But good housing is expensive. They needed safe spacious outdoor space; fresh air and exercise are valued by mothers for children's health. But living in an area with safe open space is also expensive. They needed the company of other children, but if the mother had a poor social network, company was available only through groups such as toddler groups, playgroups and nurseries, which again had to be paid for. Most of the women in this study thought good food, housing, neighbourhoods and child care directly affected their children's health and well-being. They were not extras. So, for many mothers, earning money to resource the household was intrinsic to good child-rearing.

However, social policies inhibited mothers' working behaviour. The absence of adequate nursery care prevented some mothers from working. The long hours expected of paid workers conflicted with mothers' wish to spend time with their children. They needed childcare services and employment opportunities that recognized parental responsibilities both to do paid work and to give the child parental care.

The perspectives outlined above were common to most of the mothers, whatever their background and education. The exceptions, ideologically, were the four indigenous white working-class mothers, all of whom lived with their child's father, and were content to be full-time mothers at home.

Health visitors

In contrast, almost all the health visitors thought that, ideally, mothers should be full-time carers of their children. They were seen to have many tasks: building strong affectional bonds with their children, controlling them, and stimulating their learning. However, health visitors recognized that in reality many mothers have to go out to work, either for money or to maintain their mental health. If so, they suggested that individual care by a childminder could provide the child with an adequate emotional basis for good emotional development. Only a few health visitors (4 of 28) had similar perspectives to most of the mothers: that material resources were intrinsic to good child care.

For health visitors the psychological work of mothering was the critical work, together with the physical and management work. Though they recognized that many mothers were constrained by their poor circumstances, and that mothers' own mental health suffered in consequence, most thought that with good motivation, and with support from health professionals, mothers should be able to give their children good care, whatever their material circumstances.

Knowledge and intervention

Mothers

The foregoing sections have suggested some major sources of mothers' and health visitors' knowledge of childhood and child care. Where does this knowledge come from? Mothers' knowledge was experiential. They learned how to care for their child through experience and, in the course of this caring experience, they learned what aspects of their material and social environment mattered for the child's health, progress and well-being. Apart from this experiential knowledge, mothers had a wide range of sources of knowledge. They learned from other mothers, especially from their own mothers and sisters, but also from friends with children. As in other studies, almost all of the mothers had at least one childcare book, and most had leaflets they picked up at the clinic. They also watched television programmes on child care. Many of them found health visitors and doctors useful sources of information, especially mothers who had come to the UK recently, who did not have frequent contact with their relatives, and so were particularly isolated.

Mothers assumed that it was on the basis of their knowledge, acquired from many sources, that the care of their child took place. They were the people who took the day-to-day decisions in child care! Their criteria for success were based on their own values and goals for their children. However, they also recognized the value of doctors' and health visitors' knowledge and acquired expertise, and were glad to have this professional appraisal of their child's health and progress, during meetings and at check-ups. They saw it as their own responsibility to decide whether and when to take up these services.

As suggested earlier, mothers put great emphasis on the importance of material factors in affecting the quality of the child's experiences and, indeed, on the care they could give. A secure adequate income, good housing, a pleasant neighbourhood, good local services, all critically affected the child's health and welfare. Many mothers expressed the view that society should help them by facilitating their access to a reasonable standard of living for themselves and their children.

Health visitors

Most of the health visitors drew mainly on book knowledge – especially developmental psychology – in their expressed views. As the preceding sections suggest, they were comfortable with the assumptions many such texts – and most social policies – make about motherhood and child care. Notably, those who were mothers themselves (and about half of them were) did not draw on that experience in their accounts of good child care. Professionalism overrode experience?

A distinctive feature of health visitors' expressed views was that they regarded their knowledge as factual. That is, they described their ideas about good child care and child-rearing, using words such as 'correct', 'objective' and 'right'. All except four of the health visitors referred to themselves as professionals with an objective body of knowledge, the other four arguing that the goals and methods of child care are very much a matter of opinion and moral judgement.

It was also striking that virtually no health visitors questioned the desirability of their interventions in parental child-rearing to promote their own preferred practices. It was self-evident to almost all the health visitors that mothers should use the services offered, they should attend the clinic regularly in the child's early months, and bring her for check-ups as and when the clinic offered these services. The health visitor's role here was to promote universal take-up of services.

Finally, when considering factors affecting the quality of child care, health visitors on the whole put more stress on psychological factors than on material ones. It was on the psychological front that they felt they should and could intervene to promote good child care, rather than at the wider societal or resource level.

Thoughts about the community child health services

This chapter has shown that mothers and health visitors have different perspectives on child care. These differences concern children as people or as projects, child development and the role of adults, children as sociable people, and definitions of responsible behaviour by mothers.

Mothers put a high value on their own knowledge, and felt it to be most relevant to the care of their child, but they were keen to seek more of – and appreciated being able to draw on – the knowledge and expertise of doctors and health visitors. Health visitors, however, gave a higher value to professional knowledge, which they saw as correct and objective; they saw mothers' knowledge as partial and often faulty.

Mothers were in no doubt that they were responsible for the maintenance and promotion of their children's health and welfare. However, health visitors felt responsible for improving standards of child care among 'their' mothers.

Mothers relied on their own values and goals as criteria for success in child care, but valued the opinion of health service providers, especially doctors, who had technical knowledge and experience. Health visitors assumed that the criteria for success rested on professional assessment and judgement. They held medicalized criteria for success in child care.[3]

Mothers located the causes of success or failure in child care in the material and social environment, whereas health visitors put more stress on psychological factors.

This book is being written at a time of change in thinking and practice in community child health services. Health visitors, as an occupational group, are increasingly recognizing that they must change both their goals and methods of working in the community, as regards both mothers of small children and other groups.[4] Many pioneer projects are underway;[5,6] management staff in conjunction with doctors and community nurses are developing new models for services. The data from this study cannot contribute to these debates and plans at the level of detailed suggestions for service provision. However, the differences in perspectives outlined above, deriving though they do from one small study, do provoke thought about the general framework of assumptions underpinning the provision of services.

The perspectives of health visitors who took part in this study broadly reflect the characteristics and goals of traditional community child health services. On this traditional model, services are offered on the basis that staff know best what services mothers should use. A high valuation is assigned to professional knowledge. Services are interventionist in both spirit and method: services are proffered, and staff aim for and take responsibility for achieving universal acceptance and take-up of them. The help offered is mainly at the individual level, its goal is to change mothers' behaviour and it takes the form of support and advice on child care. Health services are not planned to recognize that structural and material factors affect children's health status; or to ensure good cooperation between health services and housing, social security, day care, and social service departments.

However, another model of community child health services may be considered, based on the assumption that services should be responsive to parental perspectives. Such services would recognize and value mothers' knowledge and would provide opportunities for mothers to seek more knowledge as and when they needed it; staff would also recognize fathers as parents, and consider what services they wish for, and how these can best be provided. Services would recognize parental responsibility for child care and for using services as, for instance, the French services do.[7] Staff would seek the means to recognize in practice the importance of structural and material factors in affecting the care that mothers and fathers can and do give.

Implementation of such criteria for service provision could well result in differences between areas, depending on local conditions, and the needs and wishes of local parents, as well as of health service staff. Clinics and health centres might be open for longer or for more flexible hours, so that parents in employment – of both sexes – had good access. Released from the task of chasing up mothers, community health workers would be freed to develop, in conjunction with parents, ways of identifying and meeting parents' needs for information, for discussion of child care, in order to provide practical help and support. For example, health education initiatives might be led by local people in collaboration with staff and might proceed on egalitarian principles, rather than on the top-down model disliked by mothers.[8–10] Services might be made available at a number of venues, such as factories, schools, community centres and market stalls.

There are many interesting intiatives currently underway,[11] which cannot be examined here. But if we can recognize that mothers do not need surveillance and education, and if we accept that parents may welcome the development of promotive and preventive health services, which are both responsive and accessible, then the way is open for exciting new developments in the provision of community health care services into the 1990s.

Acknowledgements

The study *Perspectives on Child Care: Parents and Professionals* was funded by the Economic and Social Research Council, and carried out at Thomas Coram Research Unit (1985–8) by the author and Marie-Claude Foster.

References

1 Mayall, B. and Foster, M. C. (1989). *Child Health Care: Living with Children, Working for Children*. Oxford, Heinemann.
2 Mayall, B. (1990). The division of labour in early childcare – mothers and others. *Journal of Social Policy*. In press.
3 Graham, H. and Oakley, A. (1986). Competing ideologies of reproduction: Medical and maternal perspectives on pregnancy. In Currer, C. and Stacey, M. (eds), *Concepts of Health, Illness and Disease*. Leamington Spa, Berg.
4 Goodwin, S. (1988). Whither health visiting: Keynote speech. HVA Annual Study Conference, Bournemouth. Issued by the Health Visitors' Association, 50 Southwark Street, London SE1 1UN.
5 Billingham, K. (1989). 45 Cope Street: Working in partnership with parents. *Health Visitor Journal*, 62(5), 156–7.
6 Jackson, C. (1989). Wherefore to Oxfordshire? *Health Visitor Journal*, 62(5), 159–60.
7 Foster, M. C. (1988). The French puericultrice. *Children and Society*, 2(4), 319–34.
8 Lewis, J. (1986). The working class wife and mother and state intervention 1870–1918. In Lewis, J. (ed.), *Labour and Love: Women's Experience of Home and Family*. Oxford, Blackwell.

9 McIntosh, J. (1987). Interpersonal style and professional effectiveness: Some implications of a directive approach to health visiting. *Scottish Health Visitor Magazine*, 7, 6–10.

10 Foster, M. C. and Mayall, B. (1990). Health visitors as educators. *Journal of Advanced Nursing*, **15**(2), 286–92.

11 Drennan, V. (ed.) (1988). *Health Visitors and Groups*. Oxford, Heinemann.

Using health services

Chapter 6

Children with cough: who consults the doctor?

Sally Wyke, Jenny Hewison and Ian Russell

Respiratory illness is very common in children, and is a large proportion of general practitioners' paediatric caseload. In the 1981–2 National Morbidity Study,[1] 30 per cent of all consultations for children under 11 years were for respiratory disease. Many episodes of acute respiratory disease are self-limiting, and a doctor can do very little to contribute to the child's recovery. This, combined with the fact that many similar episodes are dealt with in the home,[2–4] has led to the widespread feeling in general practice that some parents who consult with respiratory illness in their children do so unnecessarily, inappropriately or for trivial reasons.[2,5] Parents with less formal education, or from working-class or unemployed backgrounds, are known to consult the doctor more often for their children (see also Chapter 8, this volume).[6] However, they are often perceived to be the worst 'offenders' as far as trivial consultation is concerned; possibly, it is thought, because they do not know how to use the service 'correctly'.

There is also evidence that the burden of respiratory illness is concentrated in the less affluent sections of society.[7] In England and Wales, children whose fathers are in occupational social class V (unskilled workers) are nearly twice as likely to die from respiratory illness as those whose fathers are in occupational social class I (professionals). Although morbidity data are more scarce, many *ad hoc* studies have shown that a similar pattern of inequality is seen in morbidity from respiratory illness.[8]

This chapter concerns both these issues. Drawing on a study of parents' consulting behaviour for a single episode of one symptomatic condition – children's cough – it investigates which groups of parents were more likely to consult their general practitioner with their child's cough; it goes on to investigate whether materially deprived children were reported as having worse coughs; and finally investigates if the severity of the cough alone explained consulting behaviour. Thus two interrelated questions are posed: Are parents with less material resources more likely to consult their general practitioner with their child's cough? And, if so, might this be explained by their children having worse coughs?

The study

The study design and methods have been described in detail elsewhere.[9,10] The study was linked to the Northern Regional Study of Standards and Performance in General Practice, a major study of standard setting in general practice, based on 65 training practices.[11]

The data were collected through home interviews with parents of children registered with 21 general practices in North-East England. These ranged from small, geographically dispersed practices in rural areas, to large inner-city practices.

As part of the Northern Regional Study, a postal questionnaire was sent to the parents of all the children registered in these practices 6 weeks before interviewing was due to take place. It asked about the prevalence of, and consultations for, five symptomatic conditions of childhood, including acute cough and recurrent wheezy chest. Ninety-one per cent of the parents responded. From the replies to this questionnaire we drew a random sample, stratified by practice, of 249 children. All these children had been reported as having had a cough in the 4 weeks before receiving the postal questionnaire; and half had been taken to the doctor with the cough. Twenty-three of these children could not be contacted and were replaced by similar children, and the parents of 234 (94 per cent) were successfully interviewed.

The interviews lasted about 1 hour and covered a number of topics. First, we asked about the social characteristics of the child and family, including the number of people in the household, the parents' employment status, occupation, educational attainment, and so on.

Secondly, parents' perceptions of the child's reported cough were investigated using questions designed to elicit the sort of information available to general practitioners through history taking (for example, how the cough sounded, how long it has lasted and how the child had reacted to the cough). To summarize the severity of each child's cough in a single measure, a scale was constructed from all characteristics of the cough elicited in the interview. The score for each of these characteristics was based on clinical experience rather than on the data collected in this study. The resulting scale took values between 0 (no evidence of cough) and 100 (most severe cough). The scale was not normally distributed (more children had less severe coughs), but became so by taking natural logarithms. We used the log scale of severity in all analyses.

Thirdly, using a set of six scenarios of respiratory ill-health in children,

Table 1 Scenarios of respiratory ill-health in children included in interview schedule

A   The child's cough has lasted 7 days and he or she has also been sick when he or she coughed

B   The child is normally well, but for the past month has been getting a tight chest and wheezy when running and has been unable to keep up with friends

C   The child's cough has lasted 3 weeks. It has not got worse, but it has not got better either. He or she has no other symptoms

D   The child has been wheezing for 24 hours, cannot go to school (playgroup), and cannot play with other children

E   The child's cough has lasted 2 days, he or she is off her food and has a slight temperature

F   The child has suddenly developed a wheeze. Breathing rapidly has become laboured and lips have changed colour to blue over a period of about 4 hours.

parents were asked whether they would consult a doctor if their child had those symptoms. These scenarios are shown in Table 1. Parental propensity to consult was measured by constructing a scenario response score from their replies. A score of 0 implied that a parent had said they would not consult a doctor for any of the scenarios, and a score of 6 that they had said they would consult a doctor for all six scenarios.

Who consulted the doctor?

Let us look first at the consultations for a child's cough. In general, parents with less material resources were more likely to have consulted their general practitioner with the cough (Table 2). Children whose fathers were not in paid employment, whose families did not own a car, who lived in rented accommodation (as compared to owning their own house), who lived with someone who was a smoker (usually a parent), and whose mother left full-time education before the age of 16, were all significantly more likely to have been taken to the doctor with their cough. Children whose fathers had left school before 16, or who were in manual occupational social classes were also more likely to be taken to the doctor with the cough, but these differences did not reach statistical significance.

Who had worse coughs?

As has been reported elsewhere,[10] parents with less material resources were also more likely to be reported as having had worse coughs (Table 3). Children whose fathers and/or mothers were not in paid employment, whose family did not have a car, who lived in rented accommodation, and whose mother left school before age 16 were reported as having significantly worse

Table 2 Association between selected social factors and the decision to consult

	Those who replied 'yes'		Those who replied 'no'		P
	n	% consulting	n	% consulting	
Father *not* employed?	49	67	185	36	***
Family has *no* car?	65	65	169	34	***
Accommodation rented?	71	61	163	34	***
Mother *not* employed?	142	52	92	28	***
Smoker in household?	114	52	120	34	**
Mother left full-time education before 16	153	47	81	33	*
Father left full-time education before 16	186	44	48	35	NS
Father's manual social class	151	46	83	37	NS

* Statistically significant at the 5 per cent level; ** 1 per cent level; *** 0.1 per cent level.

coughs. However, as with consulting, children whose fathers left school before 16, and who were in a manual occupational social class, were reported as having worse coughs, but the differences were not significant.

We have stressed throughout that the scale of severity of children's coughs is based on parental *perceptions* of the cough, i.e. parents' accounts of the cough reported in interview rather than as assessed by a physician on clinical

Table 3 Association between social factors and perceived severity of cough

	Mean of log of perceived severity of cough		t-value
	Yes	No	
Father *not* employed?	3.9	3.2	5.0***
Family has *no* car?	3.7	3.1	4.8***
Accommodation rented?	3.6	3.1	3.7***
Mother *not* employed?	3.5	3.1	3.3***
Smoker in household?	3.3	3.2	1.5
Mother left full-time education before 16	3.4	3.1	2.9**
Father left full-time education before 16	3.3	3.1	1.8
Father's manual social class	3.4	3.2	1.3

** Statistically significant at the 1 per cent level; *** 0.1 per cent level.

examination. Parents' accounts of their children's coughs can be seen as having two components: the cough as it actually was (or as it would have been assessed by a physician – the *objective* component); and their perception of the cough (the *subjective* component, likely to differ between parents). Parents who had perceived the cough to be worse than it was in reality are likely also to have exaggerated its severity during interview. There is a danger that a tendency to subconscious exaggeration of the child's cough was concentrated among the materially deprived parents in our sample. If so, the explanation for the fact that they report worse coughs could be simply that they perceived the cough to be worse, whereas a doctor may not have measured it as worse.

Fortunately, we can use the scenario response score to assess the likelihood of biased reporting by materially deprived parents, as reported elsewhere.[10] We reasoned that parents who perceived the scenarios to be severe and who therefore had a higher scenario response score, would be more likely to exaggerate the severity of their own child's cough. If so, we would have expected the mean log perceived severity to increase with each successive increase in the scenario response score. However, there was no such linear relationship between the scenario response score and the log scale of perceived severity (Table 4). We concluded, therefore, that variations in the objective severity of the child's cough were the main sources of variation in the reported severity, and that materially deprived children did indeed suffer worse coughs.

Does severity explain the decision to consult?

The fact that children of parents with less material resources were both reported as having worse coughs *and* were more likely to be taken to the doctor with the cough suggested that the severity of the cough was important in parents' decisions to consult. However, even if their child had a cough of similar severity to that of a child from a more affluent background, would parents with less material resources still be more likely to consult the doctor? Did they, for whatever reason, have a higher propensity to consult the doctor?

This was investigated using the multivariate statistical technique of logistic regression.[12,13] This technique explains the decision to consult using information about the severity of the cough and all the social factors that were

Table 4 Association between propensity to consult and perceived severity of cough

Scenario response score	1 or 2	3	4	5	6
Mean of log of perceived severity of cough	3.9	3.9	3.3	3.6	3.6

Note: Association not statistically significant (*F*-test for linear trend).

significantly associated with consulting. It sorts out the relationships between severity and the social factors, and determines which are most likely to have influenced the decision to consult, independent of relationships between all the factors.

The perceived severity of the cough proved to be highly predictive of consultation. After this factor had been taken into account, no other social variable could improve the prediction of consultation. Thus the associations between material deprivation and consulting were explained by materially deprived children having worse coughs. At any given level of severity of cough, parents with different levels of material resources were equally likely to consult the doctor: each group of parents in this study used similar criteria in making the decision to consult their doctor for their child.

Discussion

This chapter was based on a study of parents' consulting behaviour for a single symptomatic episode of childhood cough, in 21 training practices in North-East England. It has answered two interrelated questions: it found that parents with less material resources were more likely to consult their general practitioner with their child's cough, but it also found that their children had more severe coughs, and this higher severity level explained the higher level of consulting. General practitioners working in deprived areas, whether inner-city or rural, probably have higher paediatric workloads than their colleagues working in more affluent areas. This has important implications in the light of new contractual agreements which do not necessarily take this fully into account when tying remuneration to workload.

At any given level of severity, parents in different socioeconomic circumstances were equally likely to consult the doctor. This finding is important because it shows that parents with different backgrounds use similar criteria in deciding whether to consult a doctor for their children. The severity of the cough and its effects on the child are the crucial criteria, while other considerations seem to play little part. In Chapter 3, Sarah Cunningham-Burley and Una Maclean discuss how most parents understand doctors' perspectives; they are aware of constraints on doctors' time and are reluctant to 'bother the doctor' or 'waste the doctors' time'. This study also suggests that parents take considerable care in deciding whether to consult a general practitioner for their child's respiratory illness. Although the illness may be self-limiting, and seem trivial to the doctor, parents do not take the decision to consult lightly, but base it on their perception of their child's symptoms and signs.

Acknowledgements

This study was funded by an ESRC-linked studentship to the Northern Regional Study of Standards and Performance in General Practice, Health Care Research Unit,

University of Newcastle upon Tyne. We thank the general practitioners who gave us access to their patients, the parents who participated in the study, and Dr Edmund Hey who made a substantial contribution to the design of the interview schedule, and who constructed the scale of cough severity.

References

1 Royal College of General Practitioners, Office of Population Censuses and Surveys, Department of Health and Social Security (1986). *Morbidity Statistics from General Practice 1981–82: Third National Study*. London, HMSO.

2 Lau, B. W. K. (1987). Trivia in general practice. *Practitioner*, **231**, 1333–5.

3 Hannay, D. R. (1980). The 'iceberg' of illness and 'trivial' consultations. *Journal of the Royal College of General Practitioners*, **30**, 551–4.

4 Pattison, C. J., Drinkwater, C. K. and Downham, M. A. P. S. (1982). Mothers' appreciation of their children's symptoms. *Journal of the Royal College of General Practitioners*, **32**, 149–62.

5 Cartwright, A. and Anderson, R. (1981). *General Practice Revisited*. London, Tavistock.

6 Campion, P. D. and Gabriel, J. (1984). Child consultation patterns in general practice: Comparing 'high' and 'low' consulting families. *British Medical Journal*, **288**, 1426–8.

7 Office of Population Censuses and Surveys (1988). *Occupational Mortality: Childhood Supplement England and Wales 1979–80, 1982–83*. London, HMSO.

8 Blaxter, M. (1981). *The Health of the Children: A Review of Research on the Place of Health in Cycles of Disadvantage*. London, Heinemann.

9 Wyke, S., Hewison, J. and Russell, I. T. (1990). Respiratory illness in children: Who consults the doctor? *British Journal of General Practice*, **40**, 226–9.

10 Wyke, S., Hewison, J., Hey, E. N. and Russell, I. T. (forthcoming). *Acta Paediatrica Scandinavica*.

11 Irvine, D. H. *et al*. (1986). Performance review in general practice: Educational development and evaluative research in the Northern Region. In Pendleton, D. A., Schofield, T. P. C. and Marinker, M. L. (eds), *In Pursuit of Quality*, pp. 146–65. London, Royal College of General Practitioners.

12 Anderson, J. A. (1972). Separate sample logistic discrimination. *Biometrika*, **59**, 19–53.

13 Russell, I. T. and Gregson, B. A. (1981). Trainees' assessments of their trainers: Statistical analysis. In Ronalds, C., Douglas, A., Pereira Gray, D. J. and Selby, P. (eds), *Fourth National Trainee Conference*. Occasional Paper 18, pp. 73–80. London, Royal College of General Practitioners.

Chapter 7

Whether or not to consult a general practitioner: decision making by parents in a multi-ethnic inner-city area

Andy Clarke and Jenny Hewison

This chapter concerns decision making by parents in a multi-ethnic, inner-city area. On what basis do parents decide to consult the general practitioner (GP) for their children? In the project described in Chapter 6, respiratory illness consultations at practices in the North-East of England were studied, and compared with illness episodes which had not led to contacts with the doctor. It was found that although more illness episodes led to consultations in materially disadvantaged families, this increase was very largely accounted for by an increase in the reported severity of the episode of cough that the parents were describing.

However, that study covered a wide geographical area, including very rural, as well as inner-city, practices. Very few families from ethnic minority groups live in rural Northumberland or County Durham and, consequently, none were included in the study sample. The study that is the main subject of this chapter was conducted in Leeds, a city which numbers among its inhabitants families from very many different ethnic minority groups. More specifically, the study was carried out in general practices whose patient lists included Sikh families from both India and East Africa, Muslim families whose origins were in Pakistan, and Afro-Caribbean families, as well as families of white indigenous origin.

The study was carried out in three general practices. Five of the six GPs were white and indigenous (two men and three women), the other (a man) came from Bangladesh. All of these GPs were very sympathetic to the needs of minority families – a fact which needs to be borne in mind when the results of the study are being interpreted. Such sympathy is by no means universal, however, and criticisms regarding 'trivial' consultations have been extended to ethnic minority families,[1] some of whom, it is alleged, 'over-use' the NHS.

However, opinions are usually all there is to go on in this area, since very little is actually known about the health behaviour of families from different minority groups, either in primary care or in the hospital sector. The authors of a recent review article about the health of British Asians commented that 'little has been published on the use of primary care services, racism in health service delivery, quality of care, and doctor–patient communication'.[2]

The present study was an attempt to find out if there was any evidence of increased rates of consultation among ethnic minority families on behalf of their children; and then, taking the parents' perspective, to see if there were any obvious differences in the health decision making of the different family groups.

Health beliefs and illness behaviour

Very many articles and books have been written by psychologists, sociologists and anthropologists on the beliefs which people hold about health and illness, and on how they make decisions and act in different circumstances. Attempts have been made to construct theoretical models of health beliefs and behaviour, but when tested against what people actually do, their explanatory power is unimpressive. This study was designed in the knowledge of this work, but not as a test of any one theoretical model. In general terms, the guiding principle behind the study was that 'illness', as perceived by patients or their parents, may have psychological, social and cultural components to its definition, which are absent from more medically oriented definitions of 'disease'.

Parents are continually having to make complex decisions about their children's health (see Chapter 3, this volume) and doctors probably see only about 10 per cent of all the illness episodes identified by parents.[3] It also seems that when parents make their health decisions, the perceived clinical characteristics of the illness and the behaviour of the child are the most important factors in predicting what the parents will do (see also Chapter 6, this volume).[4] In the indigenous population at least, specifically subcultural or social factors seemed to be of very minor importance. Thus, it was anticipated that in the Leeds study, however many consultations there might be in the different family groups, these would reflect rational decisions made by the parents: as was noted in Chapter 6, a condition which is trivial to a doctor may not be so to the anxious parents of an ill child.

The study of consultation rates

None of the three general practices in which the study was carried out recorded the ethnic origin of families on their lists. Names were therefore used in the first instance to distinguish Asian and non-Asian families, a distinction that is commonly used in the localities where the practices were situated, but which obviously requires considerable caution for any more serious purpose. In this preliminary exercise, 'Asian' families comprised Sikhs and Pakistani Muslims, while 'non-Asians' were mainly white indigenous families and a relatively small number of Afro-Caribbeans. Using names in this way has since been shown by other health researchers to be an accurate means of ascribing Asian ethnic identity in English populations.[5]

To estimate consultation rates, all children aged between 2 and 11 years and registered with the three practices were identified from practice lists, and a record was made whenever they consulted over a specified 3-month period. Children were then classified as either 'consulters', that is, they had consulted their GP at least once during that time, or 'non-consulters', the remaining children (Table 1).

The figures in Table 1 refer to all consultations; they show that Asian families were more likely to have consulted than non-Asian families. Further analysis suggested that the increase in consultation rates seen in the Asian families was particularly marked for respiratory conditions: 58 per cent of all consultations for these illnesses were from Asian families, whereas the figure for other illnesses was only 42 per cent.

Returning to the crude distinction between Asians and non-Asians, the Sikh and Muslim families in this study tended to be registered with different general practices, because of the different areas in which they lived. The trend towards increased consultation rates among Asian families was found in practices serving both Sikh and Muslim communities, suggesting that the effect was not confined to just one of these groups.

The decision to consult

In the second part of the study, we interviewed parents of 2- to 11-year-old children who had recently consulted their GP for a respiratory illness in their child; and compared the information they gave with that from parents who had not consulted their GP for such an illness in the previous 6 months. Including pilot studies, 159 parents were interviewed in all, but most of the findings reported here come from the 107 families who took part in the main study.

The doctors in the three practices identified the 'consulters' when the families consulted about a target respiratory illness. For each consulter, a non-consulting family, matched by sex and age of child, was sought from the practice list. Criteria adopted for inclusion in the study were that the family

Table 1 Consultation rates

	Consulters	Non-consulters	Total registered
'Asian'	250	353	603
'Non-Asian'	238	553	791
Total	488	906	1394

$\chi^2 = 19.15, P < 0.001$.

had not consulted their GP for any respiratory illnesses, for any of the children in the family, over the previous 6 months.

We could not find suitable matches for all the families, and 59 consulters and 48 non-consulters were finally interviewed. It is important to note, therefore, that in the results from here on, the total numbers of families do not carry useful information in themselves: they reflect the research method chosen, not facts about the world. Few families refused when approached and asked to take part in the study – about 5 per cent of the total number contacted.

The family interviews were based on structured questionnaires, and covered five main areas. First, we asked about the sociodemographic characteristics of the family: parents' jobs and education, family composition and material circumstances.

Secondly, we asked about the severity of the target (most recent) episode of respiratory illness. We used the same set of questions as in the study described in Chapter 6: they were designed by a research paediatrician to capture the same information that a GP could gather during history taking.[6] There were questions about various signs and symptoms, their duration, and the way in which the cough affected the child. The answers were combined and weighted to produce a summary of cough severity (see Chapter 6, this volume). In this section, 'non-consulting' parents were asked about the last episode of respiratory illness suffered by the target child. Of the 48 families in this group, 13 reported that their child had had no illness of this kind during the previous 6 months, and therefore data from the 'severity' section of the interview is missing for these families.

Thirdly, using a set of eight standard scenarios of ill-health, parents were asked 'What would you do if. . . ?' The scenarios are listed in their original order in Table 2; they are similar to those used in the study described in Chapter 6. Fourthly, we asked questions about general health beliefs, seeking parents' views on the causes of coughs and colds, their appropriate home management, and likely prognosis.

The last section of the interview was devoted to questions on satisfaction with health care. A previously validated scale was used,[7] which covered:

Table 2 The scenarios of ill-health

A	The child's cough has lasted for 7 days and he or she has also been sick usually when he or she coughed
B	The child is normally well, but for the past month has been getting a tight chest and wheezy when running
C	The child's cough has lasted for 3 weeks and has not got any worse but neither has it got any better. He or she has no other symptoms
D	The child has been hot and miserable for 24 hours, drinking plenty of fluids, but refusing food
E	The child has had a runny nose and a fine rash for the last 24 hours. There are no other symptoms
F	The child has been wheezing for 24 hours, so he or she could not go to school or playgroup and he or she could not play with other children
G	The child is off his or her food and has a slight temperature, but no other symptoms
H	The child quite suddenly had difficulty breathing and his or her lips changed colour to blue in a period of about 4 hours

1 Access to the doctor, e.g. waiting times for appointments and waiting time at the surgery.
2 Satisfaction with the care given by the doctor in the consultation, e.g. how concerned the doctor seemed to be, and how much information the patient was given.
3 Satisfaction with the overall way the practice was organized, including factors such as the perceived helpfulness of the practice staff and whether or not the patient had ever had any bad experiences connected with the practice.

The interviews took about 45 minutes to conduct. Six of them were interpreted, three by an adult relative of the family and three by a professional interpreter. Five of the six were with Muslim families, and one with a Sikh family. Table 3 gives the final composition of the interview sample.

Table 3 The families in the main study by consulting behaviour and ethnic group

	Consulters	Non-consulters[a]	Total
White	20	16 (5)	36
Muslim	17	12 (3)	29
Sikh	12	12 (4)	24
Afro-Caribbean	10	8 (1)	18
Total	59	48	107

[a] Figures in parentheses refer to the numbers of families where no illness was reported for the child.

Results of the interview study

Sociodemographic factors

A large number of differences was found between the ethnic groups on the sociodemographic variables, but the *pattern* that emerged was clear: the Muslim and Afro-Caribbean families were socially, economically and environmentally disadvantaged compared to families from both the Sikh and indigenous communities. Parents in Muslim families were less likely to be in employment than in any of the other groups (fathers as well as mothers, the latter being known to have a very low rate of employment); parents in Afro-Caribbean families were more likely to have manual jobs; families in both groups were less likely to own their homes, to have central heating, or to own a car, and more likely to have damp in their house. Fifty-four per cent of the indigenous families earned more than £200 per week, compared to 40 per cent of the Sikh families, 13 per cent of the Afro-Caribbeans, and 4 per cent of the Muslims. The only environmental factor that cut across this trend of health-related disadvantage was that parents in indigenous families were more likely to smoke.

Consulting and non-consulting families showed only two differences on the sociodemographic variables: mothers who were employed, and particularly those who had manual jobs, were more likely to be consulters.

The severity of the target respiratory illness

In analysing this data, we found the concept of a severity threshold at which parents were likely to consult useful. For example, if parents from certain ethnic groups tend to consult for illnesses that are not very serious (i.e. they have a lower severity threshold for consulting), this would be reflected in a lower mean severity score for consulting families from that group.

Mean scores on the severity scale for consulters and non-consulters in the four ethnic groups are given in Table 4. Statistical analysis revealed that the illness episodes reported by consulters had much higher severity scores than those reported by non-consulters, and that this pattern was similar for all ethnic groups. There was no evidence that either of the Asian groups had a lower threshold for consulting; the trend for the Muslim families was if anything in the opposite direction.

The severity scores given in Table 4 do not themselves convey any sense of the kind of illness under discussion. To remedy this, consider these illustrations. The mean perceived severity score for non-consulters was 20, and a child with this score would have symptoms like these:

> The child, who was two years old, was kept awake for one night by a high temperature. The following day she was quite tired, vomited a couple of times, and needed more attention and comforting than usual.

Table 4 Mean of perceived severity scores (numbers of children in brackets)

	White	Muslim	Sikh	Afro-Caribbean	Total
Consulters	47.4	60.5	43.3	52.0	51.1
	(20)	(17)	(12)	(10)	(59)
Non-consulters	20.6	14.6	26.0	18.7	20.3
	(11)	(8)	(9)	(7)	(35)

> After 24 hours and some Calpol, the temperature had returned to normal and, although her regular eating habits were disturbed for a couple of days, she was much better.

An illness that produced a severity score near the mean for the *consulters* (51) might have had features like these:

> This six year old child had a chesty cough for almost two weeks. It tended to be worse during the night, and kept the child awake throughout the duration of the illness. The parents reported that they could hear wheezing on the child's chest, and although he didn't actually *need* more attention and comforting, he had become quite unwell at one point.

The scenarios of respiratory ill-health

One difficulty in interpreting the severity scores is that each parent is describing a different episode of illness. A parent who tended to worry a lot about such episodes might unknowingly exaggerate when describing the child's symptoms, and make them sound more severe than they actually were. Because in a study of this kind, no independent account is available of the child's illness, it is impossible to separate details of the *actual* episode from the characteristics of parents as reporters of illnesses in their child.

One way of trying to get around this is to present all parents with a set of 'standardized' illness episodes – that is, brief accounts of symptoms and behaviour in fictitious children – and ask if they would consult in those circumstances. If groups of parents are found to respond differently to these hypothetical scenarios of respiratory ill-health, it can be reasoned that this must reflect differences in their general approach to consulting, rather than differences in the types of illness suffered by their children. Put another way, scenarios are a way of asking: At any *given* level of severity, are some parents more likely to consult than others?

The parent groups which were compared in terms of their scenario responses were first, consulters and non-consulters with respect to the original target respiratory episode, and second, the four different ethnic groups.

When comparing one of the milder scenarios ('the child has been hot and miserable for the last 24 hours, drinking plenty of fluids but refusing food'), families from the consulting group were considerably more likely than the non-consulters to say that the child in the scenario needed to be seen by a doctor (44 *vs* 13 per cent). None of the other scenarios, nor a combined scenario score, showed a difference between the consulting and non-consulting groups.

We also found no difference in comparisons between the responses of parents from the different ethnic groups, either on individual scenarios or on the overall scenario score.

These results suggest that, at least for some milder illnesses, the decision to consult for any *particular* episode (and therefore to appear in the study's consulting or non-consulting groups) may in part reflect more *general* differences in parents' approach to consulting.

As the four ethnic groups were very similar in their responses to the scenarios, results from this part of the study do not contribute to the explanation of the increased consultation rates previously observed in the Asian groups of parents.

Parents' health beliefs

All of the parents in the Muslim, Sikh and Afro-Caribbean groups in the study had been born outside the UK, except for one Afro-Caribbean mother. People brought up in the Indian sub-continent, in East Africa and in the West Indies will undoubtedly have had different experiences of health and illness from those brought up in a city in the north of England. The 'common cold', for example, is seen as much more serious in some cultures and countries than it is in Britain.[8]

Parents were asked about their views on the causes of coughs and colds, the prognosis of such illnesses, and the best ways to manage them.

The causes of coughs and colds
When parents were asked, 'How do you think children get colds?', six main types of cause were mentioned. These are listed in Table 5, together with the percentage of parents in the four groups who mentioned each one. On all causes except 'improper clothing', clear differences emerged between the four groups, with indigenous families opting for germs and viruses, and the other groups attaching particular importance to the weather. It was also found that non-consulters were more likely than consulters (58 *vs* 34 per cent) to believe that germs and viruses caused their children's coughs and colds.

Prognosis of the cold
In order to identify health beliefs that might be directly associated with the decision to consult, parents were also asked, 'In your opinion, what would happen if you just left your child's cold alone? If you did nothing for it?' and,

Table 5 The causes of children's colds mentioned by the parents in the four ethnic groups

Cause of cold	Percentage who mentioned it				Significance[a]
	White	Muslim	Sikh	Afro-Caribbean	
Cold weather	17	69	88	50	$P < 0.001$
Germs/bugs/viruses	81	38	17	28	$P < 0.001$
Improper clothing	14	24	29	17	
Food/drink	3	0	33	6	$P = 0.001$
Weather changes	6	24	0	11	$P = 0.02$
Damp housing	6	0	4	22	$P = 0.02$

[a] Probabilities were derived from chi-square analyses.

in addition, 'Do you think they would tend to get worse, or do you think they would tend to get better on their own?'

Twenty per cent of parents gave conditional replies, such as 'It depends on which child' or 'It depends if there is an infection.' The responses of the remaining 85 families are given in Table 6, classified first by whether the family had consulted or not consulted for the original target episode, and second, by ethnic group. Families who had consulted for the original target episode of respiratory illness were more likely to hold the general belief that colds get worse if left alone; and this was true across ethnic groups. It was also found that Sikh and Muslim families were more likely than the others to hold this general belief.

Table 6 The prognosis of the common cold

	By consulting behaviour		
	Consulters	Non-consulters	Total
Worse	26	14	40
Better	18	28	46

	By ethnic group				
	White	Muslim	Sikh	Afro-Caribbean	Total
Worse	5	16	13	6	40
Better	25	7	8	6	46

The treatment of coughs and colds
When all parents were asked if they tried any of their own treatments for coughs and colds, instead of those obtainable from the doctor, 88 per cent of parents said that they did try to treat their children's colds in this way. Consulters and non-consulters gave very similar replies to this question, and so did members of all four ethnic groups.

Calpol (a proprietary brand of paracetamol suspension) was the most common remedy, used by three-quarters of indigenous families, half of Sikh and Muslim families, and a quarter of Afro-Caribbean families. The preferred treatments of the last mentioned group were herbal remedies and honey and lemon mixtures. When asked explicitly about coughs, parents replied slightly differently, as shown in Table 7. Cough mixture bought from a shop was easily the most common treatment overall. It was used least by Sikh families who relied extensively on herbal remedies, especially herbal teas:

> Well . . . cardomens, cloves, mint, aniseed. . . . I would make up a similar tea if they were sick as well. We use many herbs for their illnesses. Also, dry ginger tea with aniseed is good for bad colds. It's easy to do because we have it all at home.

An important belief the parents did have about these remedies was they were not seen as cures – only 4 per cent of parents saw them as such. The large majority saw them as a way of easing symptoms and helping the child sleep at night. In the words of one parent, this put the child in 'a stronger position from which to fight the illness'.

Fourteen per cent of the parents who used cough mixture did not believe that it even helped the symptoms. Explanations varied, but a common response was that it was harmless, and they were seen by their child to be doing something:

> I use Buttercup Syrup® for tickly coughs. It makes them feel easier. But I'm not sure that these cough mixtures actually do any good. They think I'm doing something for them, so I suppose in that way it helps.

Table 7 The percentage of parents in each ethnic group who used the main 'home remedies' for coughs

	White	*Muslim*	*Sikh*	*Afro-Caribbean*	*Significance*[a]
Cough mixture	79	80	44	67	$P < 0.05$
Honey and lemon	17	5	11	40	$P < 0.075$
Herbal	8	10	44	27	$P < 0.025$
Vick (a vapour rub)	8	10	0	0	

[a] Probabilities were derived from chi-square analyses.

What did parents expect to get from the doctor?
The parents were asked, 'In your opinion, what is the most important thing to receive from the doctor when you take your child with a cough or a cold?' There were three main kinds of response: antibiotics, reassurance, and other medicine (which was described in various ways). The most common response, given by exactly half the families, was that reassurance was the most important thing to receive from the doctor. Contrary to a popular myth among health care providers, fewer than 20 per cent of families mentioned antibiotics in reply to this question.

Table 8 shows the number of families giving the different responses, classified first by whether or not the family was a consulter for the target episode, and second, by ethnic group. Families who had, and had not, consulted for the target episode showed very different patterns of replies to this question, with non-consulters exhibiting a clear preference for reassurance that was not apparent in the other group. White indigenous parents were most likely to go for reassurance, and least likely to mention that it was some other medicine that they usually wanted from the doctor.

Analysing these two factors together, it appeared that if a parent believed that a medicine was the most important thing to receive from the doctor, then that parent was more likely to consult for a particular target episode; furthermore, that Asian families – particularly the Pakistani Muslims – were more likely than the other groups to hold that belief. In the words of one Pakistani mother, when asked the most important thing to receive from the doctor, 'Just a good medicine really. They seem to know what to do. They're good doctors.'

Table 8 The most important thing to receive from the doctor

	By consulting behaviour		
	Consulters	Non-consulters	Total
Antibiotics	10	9	19
Reassurance	21	31	52
Other medicine	27	7	34

	By ethnic group				
	White	Muslim	Sikh	Afro-Caribbean	Total
Antibiotics	8	8	2	1	19
Reassurance	21	7	13	11	52
Other medicine	7	12	9	6	34

Parental satisfaction with the children's health care

Access to care
This measure included ease of getting appointments and waiting time in the surgery. Families who had and had not consulted for the original target episode showed very similar, and very high, levels of satisfaction. In both the consulting and non-consulting groups, however, there were differences in satisfaction level between the ethnic groups, with Muslim families being the least satisfied and Sikh families the most satisifed in each case.

Interaction with the doctor
This measure concerned parents' satisfaction with the way the doctor interacted with both the child and parents. No differences were observed on this measure between consulting and non-consulting families; but again, there were differences between the ethnic groups. This time the indigenous families were most satisfied, closely followed by the Sikhs. Afro-Caribbean families were least satisfied, in both the consulting and non-consulting groups.

The practice as a whole
This third measure, which included whether the parents had had any bad experience at the practice as a whole, and the care given by everyone who worked at the practice, did not reveal any differences between groups.

Discussion

Taking the results of the study as a whole, it seems that the Asian parents in our sample did consult at a slightly higher rate than their indigenous or Afro-Caribbean counterparts. However, the mean severity of the illness episodes described by consulters did not differ significantly across the four ethnic groups, and so a simple explanation in terms of a lower perceived severity threshold for consulting seems unlikely to be adequate. It might be that in the practices as a whole, *more* Asian children have episodes of illness severe enough to reach consultation threshold; this would be compatible with a higher rate of consultation among Asian families, *and* a similar average level of severity among consulters.

The research design used in the present study unfortunately did not permit this possibility to be tested. The explanation is a plausible one as far as the Muslim children are concerned, because the physical and economic disadvantage suffered by many of the Muslim families in the study was quite likely to be associated with higher rates of ill-health in their children. A different explanation would, however, have to be found for the Sikhs, who were not materially disadvantaged when compared to other study families.

Although overall, consulters had higher mean severity scores than non-consulters, there was quite a lot of variability *within* each of the groups, and the severity scores of consulters and non-consulters did overlap. Additional explanations are therefore required as to why, at a given level of severity, some families did consult and others did not.

We did find that parents' health beliefs seemed to contribute to the decision to consult, over and beyond the severity of a particular episode. Parents who were pessimistic about the prognosis of an untreated cold were more likely to consult their doctor, as were parents who chose medicine rather than reassurance when asked what they wanted the doctor to provide. Asian parents were more likely to believe both these things and it is possible that these and similar beliefs may have contributed to the increased consultation rates among Asian families observed in the earlier part of the study.

Further, parents known to have consulted for the study's target episode were more likely to think a consultation was required when asked to make a decision about a mild illness described in a scenario, but this did not differ between ethnic groups.

Scores on the measures of satisfaction with health care, while showing some interesting and important differences between ethnic groups, were not apparently related to the decision to consult, at least in this fairly satisfied sample. This is worthy of comment. The GPs who took part in the study were anxious to deliver a good service to *all* of their patients. They were concerned to understand different points of view, and to explain to parents their reasons for managing childhood illness episodes in particular ways. Even in these very special and sympathetic practices, there was a substantial gulf of understanding between the doctors and at least some of their patient groups. The position in the average, still less the below average, general practice can only be a matter for speculation.

Certain factors were, of course, beyond the doctors' control. Despite the efforts which some had made to learn the basics of relevant Asian languages, they had not acquired sufficient fluency to conduct any kind of extended discussion in those languages. Because many of the mothers in the Muslim families in particular had themselves an imperfect understanding of English, communication difficulties presumably made 'reassurance' rather less meaningful for them than for English speakers. Perhaps this made the receiving of a prescription more attractive in consequence because it was something tangible, something to be taken away.

It also seems likely that ordinary coughs and colds have different significance and meaning for some families than for others. The typical white British-born family is highly familiar with such episodes, and their time course and natural history in the context of the typical British climate. It seems both probable and understandable that not all families share this lack of threat when confronted with respiratory illness in their children.

As in the study reported in Chapter 6, the severity of the particular illness episode seems to have been the factor which had most influence on whether or not the parent decided to consult. That said, at any given level of severity, parents' beliefs about the nature and likely outcome of coughs and colds probably contributed to their decision making; and Asian families did seem to hold the more pessimistic views.

Such cultural and subcultural differences are unlikely to remain constant over time, as children growing up in this country become parents in their turn. For the present, it would seem to be in both patients' and doctors' interests that the differences be acknowledged and responded to sympathetically. Information and advice tailored to parents' specific concerns are more likely to reduce anxiety levels, and help parents make the difficult decision as to whether or not a consultation is needed for any particular episode of childhood illness.

Acknowledgements

This study was funded by an ESRC-linked award to the Northern Regional Study of Standards and Performance in General Practice. We would like to thank the GPs and parents who took part in the study.

References

1 Wright, C. M. (1983). Language and communication problems in an Asian community. *Journal of the Royal College of General Practitioners*, 33, 101–4.

2 Ahmad, W. I. V., Kernohan, E. E. M. and Baker, M. R. (1989). Health of British Asians: A research review. *Community Medicine*, 11, 49–56.

3 Spencer, N. J. (1984). Parents' recognition of the ill child. In MacFarlane, J. A. (ed.), *Progress in Child Health*, Vol. 1. Edinburgh, Churchill Livingstone.

4 Wyke, S., Hewison, J. and Russell, I. T. (1990). Respiratory illness in children: Who consults the doctor? *British Journal of General Practice*, 40, 226–9.

5 Nicoll, A., Bassett, K. and Ulijaszek, S. J. (1986). What's in a name? Accuracy of using surnames and forenames in ascribing Asian ethnic identity in English populations. *Journal of Epidemiology and Community Health*, 40, 364–8.

6 Wyke, S., Hewison, J., Hey, E. N. and Russell, I. T. (forthcoming). Respiratory illness in children: Do deprived children have worse coughs? *Acta Paediatrica Scandinavica*.

7 Zastowny, T. R., Roghman, K. J. and Hengst, A. (1983). Satisfaction with medical care: Replications and theoretic re-evaluation. *Medical Care*, 21, 294–322.

8 Harwood, A. (1971). The hot–cold theory of disease. Implications for treatment of Puerto Rican patients. *Journal of the American Medical Association*, 216(7), 1153–8.

Chapter 8

'Appropriate' use of child health services in East London: ethnic similarities and differences

Elizabeth Watson

Poor or 'inappropriate' use of health care services by parents for their children has been implicated as an exacerbating factor in 'preventable' infant deaths and in causing serious childhood illness.[1-4] A knowledge of parental perspectives of the services provided is essential if reasons for this poor or 'inappropriate' uptake of services are to be understood. A number of research projects concerning parents' (usually mothers') attitudes to and use of child health services emerged in the 1980s,[5-9] and this volume is designed to make the results of some of this research more widely available (see especially Chapters 3–7, this volume). Nevertheless, particular misgivings have recently been expressed about the delivery of infant health services in the inner city[10,11] and there remains relatively little information on parents' needs and aspirations for these services in this setting.

This chapter reports on a study designed to find out just that information: it investigated the use made of primary, community and hospital services in the inner city by mothers of infants in their first year of life.

The study

The study was carried out in the Tower Hamlets District Health Authority area in East London. A random sample of 101 mothers was obtained from the Notifications of Births held in the health district; six cases were selected each week until the requisite total had been obtained. A letter was sent to each mother in the sample to explain the research and to ask whether she would be prepared to take part; only four mothers refused. The mothers were interviewed in their homes by the author, with an interpreter if necessary, when their babies were 8 weeks, 8 months and 14 months old.[12] A tape-recorder was used as a back-up to clarify any ambiguities. (Two mothers refused to be taped, although they were happy to be interviewed.)

The interviews

The first interview, when the child was 8 weeks old, focused on the professional care the women received during the antenatal, delivery and post-natal periods. It also included questions on the health of both mother and child, the use of health services, and questions about socioeconomic circumstances that might influence health.

The second interview, at 8 months, focused on the take-up of preventive child health services since the 8 week visit, and the mothers' attitudes to them.

The third interview, at 14 months, concentrated on the health care received by the children in relation to their health, and on the mothers' levels of satisfaction with the services offered. In addition, some of the questions asked at the first two interviews were repeated to provide comparative data.

The mothers

Tower Hamlets Health District serves a large, heterogeneous and multi-ethnic population, and the study sample reflected this diversity. It included 49 indigenous women (with at least two generations domiciled in the UK), 28 Bengali women, 12 West Indian women, and the rest were Sikh, Indian, Chinese, Egyptian, Vietnamese or Greek. It was useful to compare the views and experiences of women in different ethnic groups and, for the purpose of analysis, the mothers were split into three groups: non-English-speaking (who were all Bengali speakers); those who spoke English but were not born in the UK (here called English-speaking immigrants); and an indigenous group.

The Bengali women

Most Bengali women in Tower Hamlets come from the rural district of Sylhet in Bangladesh and have settled in the small decaying area of Spitalfields, in or around the notorious Brick Lane. Very few live outside this locality for well-founded fears of harassment. Although sharing certain characteristics with other Asian cultures, the Bengalis have their own distinct background, religion and culture.

Schooling is not obligatory in Bangladesh and there is a high rate of illiteracy, although many of the young mothers in the sample could read.

Most Bengalis are Muslim and adhere strictly to the tenets of the Islamic religion. In Islam, the institution of the family is sacrosanct. Often comprising a group of three or more generations, it extends its duties and obligations beyond the Western concept of the family. This pattern is followed in Britain with the paternal grandmother playing a dominant role when she lives with the family. Free mixing of the sexes is generally disapproved of, except within the family, and the woman's role outside the home is severely restricted.

The English-speaking immigrant women

This was a heterogeneous group with the largest number being, in the main, West Indian single parents with little support from their families. One Egyptian and one Indian mother did not have close family ties in the UK either, but the other women in this group had relatives near at hand. All, apart from one Chinese woman, could speak English well.

The indigenous women

Despite tower block development and reported isolation of the 'nuclear family', the realities for most of the indigenous families living in East London accorded closely to Young and Wilmot's findings in the 1950s of close kinship ties.[13] Most of the young people had one or both sets of parents living in the vicinity with 'her' mother helping the couple. They felt extremely strong ties with their own particular neighbourhoods – the 'Island' folk, Bow or Mile End populations – and all young mothers felt firm allegiance. Those in tower blocks did complain about lifts that were often out of service and about vandalism in the corridors. There were complaints too about the lack of safety in the streets and caution about going out alone, but none the less they managed to maintain links with their families. Two of the sample mothers were attacked in the streets during the course of the study.

Socioeconomic circumstances

The parents

Table 1 summarizes the study families' socioeconomic circumstances. On average, the Bengali mothers were younger than the other two groups. Most of the Bengali fathers worked in factories or catering and generally were in less skilled occupations than the other groups, although the number unemployed was similar to the indigenous group (11 and 9 per cent, respectively). None of the Bengali mothers was employed before or after marriage; in contrast, 44 per cent of the English-speaking immigrant women and 45 per cent of the indigenous women worked even during pregnancy. Far

Table 1 Socioeconomic circumstances of study families

	Bengali (n = 28)		English-speaking immigrant (n = 24)		Indigenous (n = 49)	
	Mother	Father	Mother	Father	Mother	Father
Mean age	23	29	25	30	26	28
Social class (%)						
1 and 2	0	4	21	32	14	12
3	0	11	37	36	45	50
4 and 5	0	74	25	9	31	27
Not employed (%)	100	11	17	23	10	10
Fully educated in UK (%)	4	18	54	41	94	94
Left school age (%)						
No school	13	0	0	0	0	0
<14	50	32	8	0	0	0
14–16	33	56	46	58	88	91
16–18	4	12	25	5	8	0
>18	0	0	21	37	4	9

fewer of the Bengali and English-speaking immigrant women had been educated in the UK compared to the indigenous women, and a significant number had left school under the age of 14.

Housing

None of the Bengali families had the use of a whole house; they were more likely to live in single rooms, usually of poor quality and rented from the private sector (Table 2). Some of this private accommodation, particularly around the Brick Lane area, seemed almost uninhabitable. The area is still redolent of Hogarth's London.

A similar proportion of all three groups were living in local authority housing (82 per cent of the Bengali women, 94 per cent of the English-speaking immigrant women and 84 per cent of the indigenous women), but there was wide variation in the type and quality of this housing. It ranged from modern, centrally heated flats and houses to old, damp buildings in a poor state of repair, often housing several generations in the same flat. A few of the indigenous women lived in sub-standard local authority flats but they were all young, co-habiting and usually squatting. More of the Bengalis were likely to share kitchens or bathrooms than the other two groups. They were less likely to have hot water, vacuum cleaners or refrigerators, and no Bengali mother owned a washing machine, although one woman had access to a shared one.

Table 2 Types of accommodation (percentages)

	Bengali (n = 28)	English-speaking immigrants (n = 24)	Indigenous (n = 49)
Whole house	0	8	14
Flat (self-contained)	67	71	80
Furnished rooms	4	0	2
Unfurnished rooms	11	0	0
Living with parents or relatives	18	21	4

The differences between the Bengalis and the other groups in respect of social factors were statistically significant, being particularly marked in respect of employment, education and facilities. All these factors undoubtedly contributed to the morbidity and subsequent use of child health services by the study mothers for their infants.

Antenatal care

The Bengali women tended to consult their doctor about their pregnancies later than the other women. The indigenous and English-speaking immigrant women were more likely to have experienced shared care. The Bengali women reported much longer waiting times in the antenatal clinic than the other two groups, some saying that they waited more than 6 hours.

Nevertheless, 82 per cent of the Bengali women said they felt that the standard of care they had received in the antenatal clinic was excellent or good, compared to only 71 per cent of the English-speaking immigrant women and 64 per cent of the indigenous women. The indigenous and English-speaking immigrant mothers' complaints centred around lack of cleanliness, impatience and lack of understanding by staff, a 'cattle market' atmosphere or 'conveyor belt' system. The Bengali women who were dissatisfied complained that appointments were all at the same time and that they could not communicate with the staff.

Only 8 per cent of the Bengali mothers went to antenatal classes and none to any form of parentcraft, most saying that they did not know of their existence. Thirty-five per cent of the English-speaking immigrant women and 56 per cent of the indigenous women went to these classes. Bengali women were less likely to see the relevance of check-ups than the other groups (for example, one said 'In Bangladesh we don't bother. We never need a doctor'), and some confessed to being worried by them (one said 'Important but I feel shy').

A higher proportion of the Bengali and English-speaking immigrant women had Caesarian sections than the indigenous mothers (14, 17 and 4 per cent, respectively). Seventy-seven per cent of the Bengali women had their husbands present at the birth, which represents a sharp contrast to the customary practice in Bangladesh where childbirth is conducted in the presence of women only.

Health of the babies

At 8 weeks

By 8 weeks, the babies had already had a large number of symptoms, although the English-speaking immigrant women's babies were reported to be the healthiest (Table 3). The Bengali children were more likely to be suffering from sticky eyes and coughs than the other babies. In the 'other' category, thrush, diarrhoea and colic were the most commonly mentioned, thrush being particularly remarked on by the indigenous population.

At 8 months

By the time of the second visit to the families, nearly half the children had had severe (as reported by the mothers) coughs and colds. The Bengali children were also reported as having had severe diarrhoea, vomiting, infectious illnesses, thrush and 'other' illnesses. For the Bengali children, this 'other' category included cysts, severe reactions after immunization, nappy rash, swelling on the head and ear trouble. For the children of English-speaking immigrant women, it included sticky eyes, impetigo and eczema. Finally, for the children of indigenous women, it included sticky eyes, nappy rash, and two falls (out of pram and pushchair).

Table 3 Symptoms in children at 8 weeks interview (percentages)

	Bengali	English-speaking immigrants	Indigenous
	(n = 28)	(n = 24)	(n = 49)
Sticky eye	36	17	24
Cough	29	17	18
Cold	39	38	22
Constipation	18	4	2
Excessive crying	4	4	2
Odd breathing	4	0	2
'Other' problems	18	18	49

Note: 28 Bengali children had 41 symptoms; 24 English-speaking immigrants had 24 symptoms; 49 indigenous children had 67 symptoms.

The Bengali and the English-speaking immigrant mothers reported their babies as having had an average of five illnesses, while the indigenous mothers reported an average of four.

At 14 months

Each group of women reported their babies as having had an average of three sets of symptoms between the ages of 8 and 14 months. However, the Bengali women reported their babies as having had more severe symptoms than the other two groups. They were reported as having had more severe coughs and colds and more than half the babies were reported as having had severe feverishness.

Contact with the general practitioner

At 8 weeks

A high proportion of the mothers had seen their general practitioners (GPs) for themselves or their babies by the time of the first interview when the children were 8 weeks old (Table 4). In addition, the Bengali mothers probably under-reported the number of GP contacts, as their husbands often collected medicine for the children.

There were very few home consultations: although a number of the women had requested these, they had been asked to bring their babies to the surgery. Fewer Bengali mothers made appointments to see their GPs compared to the other two groups, but this was because the practices they attended usually had drop-in surgeries. Perhaps as a consequence, the Bengali mothers were more likely to think they waited too long to see their GPs than the other two groups.

The Bengali mothers valued a doctor who could speak Bengali, and many of them went to the same group practice where all the doctors were Bengali; this meant that they travelled further than the other two groups, often by taxi. The indigenous and English-speaking immigrant mothers went to a diversity of general practices from single-handed practitioner to large group practices in health centres.

At this stage, all three groups were highly satisfied with their GPs (82 per cent Bengali, 92 per cent English-speaking immigrant and 81 per cent indigenous mothers were extremely satisfied or satisfied). As stated, the Bengali mothers valued being able to speak their own language with their doctors, although one Bengali woman said she liked her English doctor because his medicine worked! Often the husband had visited the doctor when the baby was ill and collected medicine without the baby having been seen. In contrast, the English-speaking immigrant and the indigenous women prized

Table 4 Proportion of mothers who saw their GPs by age 8 weeks (percentages)

	Bengali	English-speaking immigrants	Indigenous
	(n = 28)	*(n = 24)*	*(n = 49)*
For self	28	17	14
For baby	35	37	33
For both	29	25	35
For neither	18	21	18

personal relationships: 'Father figure knows what he is talking about'; 'He is friendly and will sit and listen. He is very good with children'; 'I look on her as a friend. Her husband brought me into the world.'

Where there were complaints, both the Bengali and the English-speaking immigrant women complained mainly of waiting time and lack of attention to problems: 'He gives prescription before I tell him the problem'; 'Takes no time and is rude.' The indigenous mothers had more florid complaints: 'He refuses to visit. The doctor sent a request for me to visit him for my postnatal on an old betting slip and I refused to go'; 'I called an emergency doctor in because I was bleeding. My doctor was angry and said I should not have done so because he had to pay for it.'

At 8 months

At 8 months, 98 per cent of the mothers had seen their GP with their babies since the first interview. They were all more likely to see their GP at the surgery, but more of the indigenous mothers had received home visits. The Bengali mothers reported going to their GP for their children far more often than the other two groups; the indigenous mothers were more likely to have adopted a 'wait and see' attitude. The Bengali mothers were more likely to have received medicines for their children than the other two groups, *possibly* because of their treatment expectations. It was certainly true to say that the Bengali women valued medicine highly. At an interview in one household, there were four bottles of identical medicine prescribed for the same illness and a total of 30 bottles of medicine on the same family's mantlepiece. The Bengali mothers reported going to their GP several times with the same illness, and many went weekly. There were still complaints at this interview that the doctors would not readily visit, particularly from the Bengali mothers who were also less likely to see the same GP when they went to the surgery. Nevertheless, among all the mothers there was a substantial appreciation of their GP's care.

At 14 months

Ninety-four per cent of mothers had seen their GP for their children in the 6 months since the last interview, the majority of the mothers having visited their doctors many times. One child, born to a Bengali mother, had had a continuous cold during the last 6 months and had been taken to the doctor 15 times. Another had been taken 10 times. Asked how many times they had been to their GP over the last year for their children, the Bengali mothers reported nearly twice as many visits as the indigenous mothers, and more than twice the number of English-speaking immigrant mothers (Table 5).

By the third visit, 16 women had changed their GP since the last visit: 1 Bengali woman, 6 English-speaking immigrant women, and 9 indigenous women. Nevertheless, 89 per cent of the Bengalis, 62 per cent of the English-speaking immigrants and 80 per cent of the indigenous women reported that they were either extremely satisfied or satisfied with their doctors (including satisfaction when the mothers had changed their doctors).

For Bengali women, dissatisfaction hinged around the queues and great crowds in the waiting room; for the English-speaking immigrant women, around communication problems (e.g. 'no advice, only pills'); and for the indigenous women because they could not 'sit and talk'. ('Writing a prescription as soon as you go in is not good enough. He should *listen*.')

By interviewing the mothers at length over the year it became obvious that not only did the standard of practice vary widely in the inner city, but that many parents had different expectations of good care than their GPs. One of the most respected GPs in the district was valued for his willingness to visit and 'explain things' and to examine the babies, but several mothers were concerned that he would not prescribe medicines and that therefore they had to buy patent medicines from the chemist. Prescribing was considered an important feature in general practice for all the mothers and for the Bengali mothers an *essential* component of the consultation.

It was noteworthy that throughout the three interviews, the individual solo practitioner was valued more than the practice team. It may well be that this remains the idealized GP concept for many patients, and that continuity of care is valued among mothers for their children.

Accident and emergency

At 8 weeks

A surprisingly high number of children had already been taken to Accident and Emergency Departments by the time they were 8 weeks old, and a number had been admitted (Table 6). The Bengali women's babies had been admitted for diarrhoea and one for a hernia, the English-speaking immigrant women's babies for a fall and feeding problems and the indigenous women's babies for whooping cough, respiratory infections and breathing problems.

Table 5 Mean numbers of surgery visits in last year for the baby

Bengali	English-speaking immigrants	Indigenous
13	6	8

At 8 months

Between 8 weeks and 8 months, 31 per cent of Bengali women, 19 per cent of English-speaking immigrant women, and 18 per cent of indigenous women had taken their babies to the Accident and Emergency Department when they were ill, and a number of children had been admitted. Examples of reasons for visits by Bengali women were: baby diarrhoea and vomiting (admitted to hospital); reaction to immunization (admitted to hospital); a cough and cold (GP's half-day). Examples of reasons for visits by English-speaking immigrant women were: baby had sticky eyes and constipation (admitted to hospital); baby bringing back food. Examples of reasons for visits by indigenous women were: baby fell out of pram; baby cough and temperature; baby constantly crying (admitted to hospital); baby suspected blockage (admitted to hospital).

The mothers seemed to make their own assessment of the severity of their children's illness and perceived the hospital as more suitable for 'serious' complaints and as providing a more immediate service than the GP, although many of the sick children could have been treated by the GP.

At 14 months

Again a large number of the mothers had visited the Accident and Emergency Department for their children and a substantial number had been admitted. In particular, more of the indigenous children had had treatment than was reported at the previous interviews. The Bengali children again went mainly

Table 6 Proportion of mothers using Accident and Emergency Departments by age 8 weeks (percentages)

	Bengali (n = 28)	English-speaking immigrants (n = 24)	Indigenous (n = 49)
Visited A&E dept.	11	13	25
Baby had been admitted to hospital	11	4	16

for diarrhoea, vomiting and feverishness and were considered ill enough to be admitted in several cases. The mothers of indigenous children were much more likely to go to the hospital for accidents (in eight cases), although several also went for feverishness which necessitated admission, sometimes after previously seeing the GP.

Community services

At 8 weeks

By the time the babies were 8 weeks old, health visitors had made an average of three visits to each of the Bengali and English-speaking immigrant mothers, and two visits to the indigenous mothers. Eighty-six per cent of the Bengali mothers valued health visitors' advice on feeding practices, compared to only 63 per cent of the English-speaking immigrant mothers and 39 per cent of the indigenous mothers. Most of the Bengali mothers found other aspects of health visitors' advice very helpful. There was some dissatisfaction with the service, expressed mainly by the indigenous mothers, based largely either on what the mothers regarded as the health visitors' lack of experience with young children or on their perceived interference. The mothers who complained were either those buttressed by family support and coping well, or young unmarried women who saw health visitors as authoritarian.

All the mothers had visited the child health clinic: the Bengali mothers had made an average of two visits and the English-speaking immigrant mothers and the indigenous mothers an average of three visits. Favourable comments on the clinic were made by the majority of the Bengali and the English-speaking immigrant women and half of the indigenous mothers. The Bengali women appreciated the advice, the presence of the interpreter and check-ups by the doctor, whereas the other two groups stressed the social aspects of the visit, saying such things as: 'Nice friendly place. Meet other mums' and 'Friendly staff. I know them all.'

The few Bengali mothers who did not like going to the clinic complained mainly of waiting time and not being given prescriptions which, for them, was an important component in medical care. The indigenous mothers complained of the lack of cleanliness and privacy, and of unwanted advice: 'They told me to give rusks. I prefer my mum's advice.'

At 8 months

Fifty-one per cent of the indigenous mothers said they had not seen the health visitor since their baby was 8 weeks old. The Bengali mothers had received more visits than the others; 43 per cent had seen the health visitor either fortnightly or monthly in the previous six months. Of those who had received visits, 95 per cent of the Bengali mothers, 92 per cent of the English-speaking immigrant mothers, but only 54 per cent of the indigenous mothers had found these visits helpful. The Bengali mothers stressed the importance of feeding advice and explanations about immunizations. The English-speaking immigrant mothers said they valued the chat and advice. The indigenous mothers were much more equivocal. All those who commented favourably preferred friendly older women, particularly if they had children.

A large percentage of mothers were still taking their children to the child health clinic (96 per cent of the Bengali mothers, 95 per cent of the English-speaking immigrant mothers and 88 per cent of the indigenous mothers). The main reason they went was for immunizations, although the Bengali mothers went more often for advice and treatment than the other two groups. Far more of them felt that it was still very important to go to the clinic; the majority of the indigenous mothers felt that they really only needed to visit the clinic for immunizations, a check-up and weighing, but relied on their kin for advice.

At 14 months

Fifty-four per cent of the Bengali mothers, 29 per cent of the English-speaking immigrant mothers and 40 per cent of the indigenous mothers had received at least one visit from a health visitor since the 8-month interview. The number of visits to the families ranged from 0 to 8 and it certainly seemed as if health visitors had tried to give more time to the families who had the greatest number of problems. None the less, there were families who reported no contact with health visitors, when I felt they urgently required health visitor support.

Of those who had received visits, 73 per cent of the Bengalis, 67 per cent of the English-speaking immigrant women and 50 per cent of the indigenous mothers had found them helpful. Twenty-six per cent of the indigenous mothers thought the health visitors were useless. The Bengali mothers, although nearly always saying their health visitors were helpful, would have liked more visits. The English speaking-immigrant mothers and the indigenous mothers also commented on the rarity of the health visitors' visits, the latter in particular feeling that there should be regular visiting and finding the occasional knock-on-the-door visiting practice ineffective.

The majority of the mothers were still going to the clinic, most going for weighing and developmental check-ups, although once again the Bengali mothers went more often for advice, particularly on feeding. Fewer of the Bengali mothers had completed their children's immunizations, although their initial cover had been better than the other two groups. The reasons the Bengali mothers gave for not completing their children's course of immunizations were that they had not received a card or that their babies had not been well enough to have them. It is possible that the adverse reactions to the immunizations reported at the time of the second interview had made some of them wary of having their children given further injections.

Discussion

This study followed mothers and children over a year of the children's early lives, and was concerned with their health, their use of services and their attitudes towards the services. It had all the advantages of a longitudinal study,[14] and illustrated how much children's and mothers' needs for services changed in that time.

The study families lived in a variety of circumstances, but the Bengali women probably had some of the worst living circumstances, reported more illness in their children, and used various health services more than the other two groups. Earlier studies had suggested that socially deprived families made less use of health services,[15] and particularly of preventive health services,[16-18] but this was certainly not the case in this study.

The issue of 'appropriate' use depends very much on whether one is taking mothers' or health professionals' perspectives (see Chapters 6 and 7, this volume). The issue is a complicated one to resolve: on the one hand, it can cause frustration for professionals, whereas on the other, make parents wary and uneasy about asking for advice in caring for the health of their children (see Chapter 3, this volume).

Bengali women were the most socially deprived members of the sample and they consulted their GPs more often than other women for their children. They also reported more episodes of illness in their children and each episode was more likely to be considered serious. Their increased service use was probably at least partly due to their children's increased morbidity. A contributory factor might have been their own stress, which has been seen to play a role in increasing symptom sensitivity and also in increasing the likelihood that the individual will seek professional medical care.[19] The Bengali women might also have had a higher expectation of the ability of doctors to make their children well through giving medicine: it was seen earlier that a prescription for medicine was perceived as an essential component of a consultation for most Bengali women. These women used Accident and Emergency Departments for symptoms in their children usually considered more appropriate to general practice, and although their babies were sometimes considered ill enough to be admitted to hospital, this type of use of Accident and Emergency Departments could lead to resentment among staff.

Whether or not preventive services were used 'appropriately' by mothers in this study is also difficult to illustrate. For example, at the first interview, Bengali mothers reported that they did not use the antenatal services as early or as regularly as the other mothers or visit the child health clinics as often. However, as the year progressed, they used the preventive services more than the other mothers, often going for advice, treatment or prescriptions. The one exception to this was their lower uptake of immunizations, but this probably related to their children's reactions to the early immunizations.

After the first 2 months of their children's lives, the indigenous mothers at first became disenchanted with the clinics and uncertain of the health visitor's role and, in a number of cases, objected to what they saw as her policing role, discussed elsewhere.[20] On the other hand, by the final interview, more of the indigenous mothers were wishing they could telephone their health visitors for small worries or that they could have more regular visits, reflecting their anxieties as their children left babyhood.

It certainly seemed as if health visitors compensated for the poor health and living circumstances of Bengali mothers by more home visiting, although there was less evidence of extra visiting to indigenous or English-speaking immigrant mothers in poor circumstances. This could have been due to the latter's greater reluctance to see the health visitors. Health visitors need a particular delicacy of approach and certainty about their own objectives for visiting these families. Possibly, there is a need for revising the criteria for automatic home visiting.

The majority of the Bengali and indigenous mothers had support for child-rearing from their families: they were not so isolated in the inner city as is often depicted, with the indigenous mothers in particular relying heavily on 'mum's advice'. This was not the case for the English-speaking immigrants, particularly the West Indian women, who were often bringing up their children relatively alone and also making fewer calls on the health services.

The mothers in poorest circumstances in this study (the Bengali women) reported the worst health in their babies. This double disadvantage might be compounded by language barriers when in contact with health professionals. The women certainly valued professional contacts conducted in Bengali (in the child health clinic and with their GPs). However, the influence of health service provision on overall child health is unclear, and it has been argued that health systems in industrialized societies are not generally successful in mitigating or preventing the problem of poverty.[21] It has been increasingly recognized that only by a massive commitment to the elimination of family and child poverty can major improvements in child health be affected.

Nevertheless, preventive and curative child health services were needed and, for the most part, highly valued by mothers in this study. Local planning, taking into account parents' needs and opinions, is increasingly recognized as the way forward for community child health services (see Chapter 4, this volume). Child health care which is a true partnership between professionals and parents can surely make some impact on improving child health in adverse conditions. We also need to evaluate new ways of working in terms of their effectiveness, efficiency, consumer acceptability and cost.[22,23]

This chapter has shown that within the context of inner-city deprivation, there is an exciting challenge for all those involved in developing district child health policies to plan for holistic services that will ensure that every city child has as good a chance as any child in the country to realize their maximum potential.

References

1 Cameron, J. M. and Watson, E. (1975). Sudden death in infancy in inner north London. *Journal of Pathology*, **117**, 55–6.
2 Morris, J. N. (1979). Social inequalities undiminished. *Lancet*, i, 87.
3 Pharoah, P. O. D. and Morris, J. N. (1979). Post neonatal mortality. *Epidemiologic Reviews*, **1**, 70–83.
4 Watson, E., Gardner, A. and Carpenter, R. G. (1981). An epidemiological and sociological study of unexpected deaths in infancy in nine areas of Southern England. II. Symptoms and patterns of care. *Medicine, Science and Law*, **21**, 89.
5 Roche, S. and Stacey, M. (1984). Overview of research on the provision and utilisation of the child health services. Review commissioned by the Department of Health and Social Security.
6 Blaxter, M. and Paterson, E. (1982). Consulting behaviour in a group of young families. *Journal of the Royal College of General Practitioners*, **32**, 657–62.
7 Biswas, B. and Sands, C. (1984). Mothers' reasons for attending a child health clinic. *Health Visitor*, **57**, 41–2.
8 Foxman, R., Moss, P., Bolland, G. and Owen, C. (1982). A consumer view of the health visit at 6 weeks postpartum. *Health Visitor*, **55**, 320–8.
9 Graham, H. (1979). Women's attitudes to the child health services. *Health Visitor*, **52**, 175–8.
10 The Acheson Report (1981). *Primary Health Care in Inner London. Report of a Study Group*. London Health Consortium, DHSS, London.
11 Royal College of General Practitioners (1981). *A Survey of Primary Care in London*. Occasional Paper No. 16. Royal College of General Practitioners, London.
12 Watson, E. (1984). Health of infants and use of health services by mothers of different ethnic groups in East London. *Community Medicine*, **6**, 127–35.
13 Young, M. and Wilmot, P. (1957). *Kinship in East London*. London, Routledge and Kegan Paul.
14 Golding, J. (1984). Britain's national cohort studies. In Macfarlane, J. A. (ed.), *Progress in Child Health*, Vol. 1. Edinburgh, Churchill Livingstone.
15 Cartwright, A. and O'Brien, M. (1979). Social class variations in health care and in the nature of general practice consultations. In Stacey, M. (ed.), *The Sociology of the NHS*. Sociological Review Monograph Vol. 22. Keele, University of Keele.
16 Ford, L. R. (1976). The community's unmet child health needs. *Public Health*, **90**, 54.
17 Zinkin, P. M. and Cose, C. A. (1976). Child health clinics and inverse care laws: Evidence from a longitudinal study of 1878 pre-school children. *British Medical Journal*, **2**, 411–13.
18 Graham, H. and McKee, J. (1979). *The First Months of Motherhood*. Monograph No. 3. Health Education Council, London.
19 McKinlay, J. B. and Dutton, D. B. (1974). Social-psychological factors affecting health services utilisation. In Madnick, M. E. (ed.), *Consumer Incentives for Health Care*. Canton, Mass., Watson Publishers International.
20 Watson, E. (1986). A mismatch of goals? *Health Visitor*, **9**, 75–7.
21 Blaxter, M. (1983). Health services as a defence against the consequence of poverty in industrialised societies. *Social Science and Medicine*, **17**(16), 1139–48.
22 Alberman, E. and Watson, E. (1985). Effectiveness, efficiency, acceptability and

costs in the preventive child health services. A first year report on a three year methological study. Unpublished report submitted to the DHSS.

23 Polnay, L. (1984). The community paediatric team – an approach to child health services in a deprived inner city area. In Macfarlane, J. A. (ed.), *Progress in Child Health*, Vol. 1. Edinburgh, Churchill Livingstone.

Section 4

Available knowledge

Chapter 9

The promotion of breast-feeding

Robert Drewett

Most of our current knowledge about the management of breastfeeding is the practical knowledge of those who are concerned with supporting and advising breastfeeding women in the community: the midwives, health visitors, lay breastfeeding counsellors and general practitioners (GPs) who help with it from day to day.

This chapter draws together some recent research on breastfeeding, and summarizes the findings. It attempts to answer three related questions: Who breastfeeds? What are the effects of breastfeeding? Why do women give up breastfeeding, and how can they be better helped to continue? Recent research does have something to offer our practitioners, though not perhaps as much as one would like.

Who breastfeeds?

It is very rare for those who start by bottle-feeding to switch to breastfeeding; but to switch from breastfeeding to bottle-feeding is common. Statistics concerning the numbers of mothers breastfeeding must therefore refer to a specified time from delivery. Much of the available information comes from three national surveys of infant feeding carried out by the Office of Population Censuses and Surveys (OPCS), the most recent in 1985. According to this survey,[1] 64 per cent of babies were breastfed in the first week of life, 55 per cent were breastfed at 1 week from delivery, and 38 per cent were breastfed at 6 weeks. However, within these summary figures there are important differences between different groups of women. Older women were more likely to breastfeed than younger women: 42 per cent of mothers under 20 years of age breastfed, whereas 86 per cent of mothers aged 30 or over did so. Women with more education and in higher social classes (in the OPCS surveys, the social class of the mother's husband or partner) were also more likely to breastfeed. Only 53 per cent of women who finished education at 16 or under breastfed their babies compared to 89 per cent of women who finished their education at 18 years or over. Eighty-seven per cent of women in class I breastfed at least once, compared with 43 per cent in class V.

Other studies have found similar results: a carefully conducted study of a representative sample of first time mothers in Leeds found that the best predictors of bottle-feeding were the age of the mother at the child's birth, and the age of the mother when she left school.[2]

The effects of breastfeeding

Breastfeeding and infectious disease

One of the most important benefits of breastfeeding to child health, internationally, is protection against diarrhoea. A recent review by Feachem and Koblinsky[3] summarized data on this from 35 studies in 14 countries. Over the first 3 months, the risk of diarrhoea was about three times as great in babies given no breast milk as in those exclusively or partially breastfed; protection continues throughout the first year, though to a lesser degree. A study of infant mortality on peninsula Malaysia[4] found that the risk of death between 1 week and 1 year of life was 2.5 times higher in bottle-fed babies than in breastfed babies when families had both toilets and piped water; but the risk of death was 5.2 times higher for bottle-fed babies when families had neither toilets nor piped water.

Breastfeeding also increases the interval between births in populations in which contraceptive methods are not readily available, partly through a direct inhibition of ovulation. The successful promotion of breastfeeding therefore has a highly desirable double effect: it both improves the survival of those children born, and increases the inter-birth interval. Because breastfeeding is also cheap, simple and does not require elaborate technology, it is of central importance to international maternal and child health.

The benefits of breastfeeding to child health in the UK, however, is more difficult to specify. It is not something that can be decided simply by reference to the presence of immunoglobulins, lactoferrin or lysozyme in breast milk. Their presence is not in question; what is in question is the extent to which they make a detectable contribution to the health of the child, in the homes in which they are living in this country. This can only be decided by studies relating type of feeding to children's health.

Data from the Child Health and Education Study were used to investigate the impact of breastfeeding on child health until the age of 5.[5] The children in the study were all born in the UK in the period 5–11 April 1970. Five years later, they were followed-up by a health visitor, who asked mothers about the duration of breastfeeding, and some details of the child's health over the last 5 years. The analysis used hospital admissions for gastroenteritis and lower-respiratory tract illnesses, and episodes of bronchitis reported by the mother, as measures of the impact of breastfeeding on child health.

The raw results did show consistent positive associations between the duration of breastfeeding and each of these measures (Table 1). We have just seen that breastfeeding is much more common in higher social classes; there is also clear evidence that children's health in the first 5 years of their life varies with the social class of their families.[6] This means that it is very important to take social class and other factors which differ between breast- and bottle-fed babies (such as maternal smoking[1]) into account when considering results like these. After adjusting for the effects of social position, smoking by the mother, birth weight, maternal age, child's sex and birth rank, the significant positive association between breastfeeding and the various measures of health disappeared in the careful analyses presented in this study.

The number of children studied was large (in excess of 13 000) and the lack of a clearly significant effect of breastfeeding on any of the health outcomes after proper statistical control is not likely to be due to an inadequately sized sample. Nor is it likely to be due to poor information on the duration of breastfeeding, which is reliably recalled by mothers even over an 8-year period.[7] However, the health measures depended on the mothers' recall of illness and hospitalization over the last 5 years, which could be uncertain, and hospitalization is not a direct measure of ill-health.

A comprehensive review of this area until 1984 was made in the Report of the Task Force on the Assessment of the Scientific Evidence Relating to Infant-feeding Practices and Infant Health,[8] and concluded that evidence of the protective effect of breastfeeding against infection was equivocal in Western countries. In 1988, a DHSS report[9] simply states that 'the clinical relationship between breast-feeding and infection in the infant in the developed world remains uncertain'. However, a recent study in Dundee[10]

Table 1 Duration of breastfeeding and children's illness (percentages)

	Never	< 1 month	1–2 months	3+ months	
Bronchitis (episodes)	18.3	17.0	15.2	13.0	(0–5 years)
Lower respiratory	1.3	0.7	0.7	0.7	(1st year)
admission	3.9	3.3	2.3	2.4	(0–5 years)
Gastroenteritis	1.8	1.2	1.0	0.6	(1st year)
admission	3.0	2.5	2.0	2.0	(0–5 years)

Data from Taylor *et al.* (1982).[5]
Notes: Bronchitis reported by the mother.
Hospital admissions for lower respiratory illness and gastroenteritis.
Each child is counted only once for each disorder.

has shown that when health outcomes are assessed carefully, there is a clear benefit to breastfed babies even after control for the important confounding variables of social class and parental smoking. In the Dundee study, 618 mothers and babies were followed up for 2 years. The babies were visited at home by health visitors at 2 weeks of age, at 1, 2, 3, 4 and 6 months, then every 3 months to 2 years of age. Type of feeding and gastrointestinal and other illnesses were recorded. After taking social class, maternal age and parental smoking into account, babies breastfed for 13 weeks or more had significantly less gastrointestinal illness than those bottle-fed from birth. Hospital admissions were also reduced. Babies breastfed for less than 13 weeks, on the other hand, had rates of gastrointestinal illness similar to those in bottle-fed babies. This study clearly shows the benefits of breastfeeding for babies in respect of gastrointestinal illness, although effects were less marked for respiratory illness.

Breastfeeding and bonding

Psychological, as well as physical, benefits are commonly attributed to breastfeeding;[11] in particular, that it improves mother–child 'bonding'. Although repeated from review to review on the benefits of breastfeeding, these claims actually have little basis in fact.

Bonding is a process of attachment of a care-giver to a baby. The term is used in the context of a theory that humans have a period after birth analogous to the critical period found in some mammals, a period in which the development of attachments is facilitated. Research relevant to the theory in humans is carefully reviewed by Lamb and Hwang[12] and by Herbert, Sluckin and Sluckin.[13]

There are three distinct claims about the relationship between bonding and breastfeeding that need to be distinguished:

1 Breastfeeding (and its duration) is a criterion for successful bonding.
2 Early separation (or its converse, increased contact between mother and baby) separately affects both bonding and the incidence or duration of breastfeeding.
3 Breastfeeding strengthens the mother–infant bond.

The first claim has no clear justification, and it is circular to argue that breastfeeding is one of the criteria for bonding, while at the same time arguing that breastfeeding strengthens it. The second claim has some justification as there is evidence that separation between mother and child at an early age may influence both bonding between mother and child and either the incidence or duration of breastfeeding, though neither of these claims is actually beyond dispute.[12]

The third claim is the strongest and is widely reiterated; but proper evidence in its favour is almost entirely absent. To provide good evidence of the effect of breastfeeding on bonding, a study would have to show differences in the behavioural indicators of bonding between breast- and bottle-fed babies, and take social class and other relevant differences between breast- and bottle-fed babies into consideration. To my knowledge, no study of the relationship between mother–child bonding and breastfeeding has ever done this.

There is some interesting evidence concerning the longer-term emotional effects of breastfeeding,[14] though these are not necessarily anything to do with bonding. Mothers of children in the Child Health and Education Study were asked to rate their children on a scale concerning antisocial behaviour, disobedience, irritability, temper tantrums, destructiveness and restlessness at age 5. Differences between breast- and bottle-fed children were found on this 'behaviour scale', but they were not consistent: children breastfed for a short period scored worse than those who were entirely bottle-fed. However, there are grave difficulties in using mothers' own accounts of their children's behaviour, because they reflect mothers' perceptions, which might be affected by all sorts of factors. As we have seen, mothers who breastfeed differ in many ways from mothers who bottle-feed, and these differences might mean they rate their children's behaviour differently too. Indeed, in a comparable analysis from the Christchurch Child Development Study,[15] differences between breast- and bottle-fed babies were considerably attenuated if teachers' rather than mothers' ratings were used; and after controlling for other factors, the significant effect of breastfeeding on behaviour disappeared.

In conclusion, there is little good evidence for a relationship between type of infant feeding and either maternal bonding to the baby or children's psychological health in the long term.

Giving up breastfeeding

Many women who start breastfeeding stop again after quite a short time: in the OPCS 1985 survey,[1] 19 per cent of mothers who started breastfeeding had stopped within 2 weeks, and 39 per cent had stopped within 6 weeks. The reasons for giving up breastfeeding are varied, but two common ones are pain and insufficient milk.

Pain

In a small study that recorded pain during breastfeeding day by day, nipple pain peaked on the second day after delivery, when over 60 per cent of women had some pain.[16] The proportion of women reporting pain then declined steadily over the first 2 weeks, though 20–25 per cent still had pain on days 15 and 30. There was very little by 2 or 3 months. Although a lot of this pain was mild, 12 of the 55 women in the sample characterized their worst pain as distressing, horrible or excruciating. Other studies of the first few days of breastfeeding show essentially the same picture.[17,18]

We know very little about the causes of nipple pain. It is obviously attributable to the sucking of the baby, but there is no clear evidence to explain why some women develop nipple pain and others do not, or its differing severity. The frequency and duration of feedings does not affect nipple pain.[18]

Research can offer little information to practitioners about the management of nipple pain; we are distinctly short of well-conducted studies. A survey of nipple pain conducted 30 years ago[17] found similar levels to studies conducted more recently; therefore, the problem has not been solved. Properly controlled trials – for example, of attempts to improve attachment – are necessary to identify the best way to manage nipple pain. Trials would not be unethical; they would be simple to design and to carry out, with readily measured outcomes.

Not enough milk

The other common reason mothers give for abandoning breastfeeding is that they do not have enough milk. There are two separate issues that need investigation here. One is to identify what the determinants of milk supply are and how they vary between women; the other is what breastfeeding mothers are actually referring to when they say that their milk supply is insufficient. This must be an inference from the babies' behaviour, as few women know how much milk they are producing.

Even in countries in which nutritional levels are much poorer than in Britain, no major effect of mothers' diets on milk production has been shown. However, milk production is widely believed to vary with the amount the baby is nursed. This relationship is an important one because, to some extent, the amount and duration of nursing is under the mothers' control. What evidence is there that increasing nursing does actually work?

Milk production is generally higher the more times a baby is nursed in a day,[19] but to my knowledge only one reasonably controlled study has demonstrated an increase in milk production with increased nursing. In this study,[20] women were put into the control group if their babies were born in July and August, and into the experimental group if their babies were born in September or October. The experimental group nursed their babies more often. The results reported showed that the mothers in the experimental group did produce more milk than those in the control group. An increase of 2.4 feeds per day 15 days after birth was associated with the additional production of 223 grams of milk. However, the randomization procedure was only partly effective, e.g. there was a large difference between the groups in birth weight.

In conclusion, research does support the generalization that increasing the frequency and amount of nursing increases milk production, but we still do not know for which women an increase in suckling is likely to work, and for which women it is not.

In extreme cases, lactation failure may be due to insufficient glandular development of the breast. Neifert, Seacat and Jobeal[21] found three cases of this in a single paediatric clinic over just a 6-month period. Insufficient nursing, inadequate sucking and failure of prolactin or oxytocin release were excluded as explanations. The failure of glandular development was associated with a lack of breast enlargement during pregnancy. This problem may underlie some cases of failure to thrive in breastfed babies.[22]

In an unselected group of 11 breastfeeding women, there was a strong association between breast enlargement during pregnancy and milk production at the end of the first week of lactation.[23] Breast enlargement during pregnancy ranged from 0 to 480 ml; and milk production ranged from 200 to 300 grams in women with no breast enlargement to 800 grams in those with greater than 400 ml. These individual differences mean that it is unlikely that all women will be equally effective at increasing milk production by increasing the number of nursing episodes.

In another study,[24] mothers were found to infer that they were not producing enough milk from babies' restlessness during or between feeds. Mothers were encouraged to increase the frequency and amount of nursing during these restless episodes, and they then lasted only a few days: 61 per cent were over in 4 days and 98 per cent in 8 days. However, whether it was increased nursing that actually led to the end of the restless episodes, or whether they would have stopped anyway, cannot be determined from the available data.

Pain and insufficient milk are two of the most common breastfeeding problems. There are others. Breastfeeding can be very rewarding, but it can be distressing too[25] and there is evidence for increased rates of minor depression or depressed mood in breastfeeding women, though the evidence is not entirely consistent across studies.[26]

Supplements

Women who are breastfeeding frequently give their babies other kinds of food in addition. Some give infant formula by bottle: in the OPCS survey, 34 per cent of breastfeeding mothers were doing so when the baby was 6 weeks old.[1] There is a striking association between giving bottles to babies in the first few weeks of life, and stopping breastfeeding altogether: only 8 per cent of mothers of babies given no bottle stopped breastfeeding within 2 weeks; 20 per cent of those given bottles occasionally at night stopped within 2 weeks; and 57 per cent of those given bottles at most feeds stopped within 2 weeks.[1]

However, in an experimental study, supplements were not found to influence the course of breastfeeding.[27] The study was conducted in two well-baby nurseries. Before the study proper began, supplementation was similar in the two nurseries (about 50 ml/infant/day). Breastfeeding rates during this pre-trial period were virtually identical, at 4 weeks and at 9 weeks. During the trial, 841 mothers were enrolled in the study. The two groups (corresponding to the two nurseries) did not differ significantly in age, education, socioeconomic status, parity, Caesarian delivery or birth weight. Supplementation was restricted in one of the two groups: in the restricted group, 63.1 per cent of babies received no supplementation, compared to 15.0 per cent in the controls. Infants in the restricted supplementation group lost significantly more weight, and therefore their supplements definitely were restricted. There was, however, no significant difference in the proportions breastfeeding at 4 weeks, and at 9 weeks they were identical (54 per cent in each group).

This is an interesting and completely unforeseen result. The authors infer that supplementation is a marker, rather than a cause of difficulty with breastfeeding. It would be useful to replicate the study because it is a model of what research in this area should be; it strikingly illustrates that an association, however persistent, does not necessarily result from a causal relationship; and its results are strikingly at odds with what we thought we knew.

Conclusions

Promoting breastfeeding is generally a sound strategy in furthering the goal of improving child health. In the UK, the gains to physical health may not be as great as in some other countries, but the evidence is accumulating that they are real.

Promoting breastfeeding can mean encouraging women to start breast-feeding, but it must also mean supporting it subsequently. Breastfeeding can be very rewarding, but it does not always run an easy course, and it is surprising that we have so few really well-designed studies on its proper management, because one of the main problems with breastfeeding is that so many women who wish to breastfeed give up so soon. I have emphasized problems with breastfeeding rather than its rewards in this chapter. This is not because I do not appreciate its rewards, but rather because I do not believe we are doing quite all we might in terms of research to make sure that its rewards can be more widely shared.

References

1 Martin, J. and White, A. (1988). *Infant Feeding 1985*. London, HMSO.
2 Wright, H. J., Walker, P. C. and Webster, J. (1983). The prediction of choice in infant feeding: A study of primipara. *Journal of the Royal College of General Practitioners*, 33, 493–7.
3 Feachem, R. C. and Koblinsky, M. A. (1984). Interventions for the control of diarrhoael diseases among young children: Promotion of breast-feeding. *Bulletin of the World Health Organization*, 62(2), 271–91.
4 Habicht, J., DaVanzo, J. and Butz, W. P. (1986). Does breast-feeding really save

lives, or are apparent benefits due to biases? *American Journal of Epidemiology*, **123**, 279–90.

5 Taylor, B., Golding, J., Wadsworth, J. and Butler, N. (1982). Breast feeding, bronchitis, and admission for lower respiratory illness and gastroenteritis during the first five years. *Lancet*, **1**, 1227–9.

6 Townsend, P. and Davidson, N. (eds) (1988). The Black Report. In *Inequalities in Health*. Harmondsworth, Penguin.

7 Vobecky, J. S., Vobecky, J. and Froda, S. (1988). The reliability of the maternal memory in a retrospective assessment of nutritional status. *Journal of Clinical Epidemiology*, **41**(3), 261–5.

8 Report on the Task Force on the Assessment of the Scientific Evidence Relating to Infant-feeding Practices and Infant Health (1984). *Paediatrics*, **74**, 579–761.

9 DHSS (1988). *Present-day Practice in Infant Feeding: Third Report*. London, HMSO.

10 Howie, P. W., Forsyth, J. S., Ogston, S. A., Clark, A. and du V. Florey, C. (1990). Protective effect of breast feeding against infection. *British Medical Journal*, **300**, 11–16.

11 Morrell, D. and Polack, M. (1982). Infancy and childhood. In *Practice: A Handbook of Primary Medical Care*. London, Kluwer Medical.

12 Lamb, M. and Hwang, C. (1982). Maternal attachment and mother–neonate bonding: A critical review. *Advances in Developmental Psychology*, **2**, 1–39.

13 Herbert, M., Sluckin, W. and Sluckin, A. (1982). Mother-to-infant bonding. *Journal of Child Psychology and Psychiatry*, **23**(3), 205–21.

14 Taylor, B. and Wadsworth, J. (1984). Breast feeding and child development at five years. *Developmental Medicine and Child Neurology*, **26**, 73–80.

15 Fergusson, D. M., Horwood, L. J. and Shannon, F. T. (1988). Breast feeding and subsequent social adjustment in six to eight year old children. *Journal of Child Psychology and Psychiatry*, **28**, 378–86.

16 Drewett, R. F., Kahn, H., Parkhurst, T. S. and Whiteley, S. (1987). Pain during breast-feeding: The first three months postpartum. *Journal of Reproductive and Infant Psychology*, **5**, 183–6.

17 Newton, N. (1952). Nipple pain and nipple damage. *Journal of Pediatrics*, **41**, 411–23.

18 Carvalho, M. de, Robertson, S. and Klaus, M. H. (1984). Does the duration and frequency of early breast-feeding affect nipple pain? *Birth*, **11**(2), 81–4.

19 Drewett, R. F., Amatayakul, K., Baum, J. D., Imong, S. M., Jackson, D. A., Ruckaopunt, S. and Woolridge, M. W. (1989). Nursing patterns and milk intake in Sanpatong. In van Hall, E. V. and Everaerd, W. (eds), *The Free Woman: Women's Health in the 1990s*. Carnford, Parthenon Publishing Group.

20 Carvalho, M. de, Robertson, S., Friedman, A. and Klaus, M. (1983). Effect of frequent breast-feeding on milk production and infant weight gain. *Pediatrics*, **72**, 307–11.

21 Neifert, M. R., Seacat, J. M. and Jobe, W. E. (1985). Lactation failure due to insufficient glandular development of the breast. *Pediatrics*, **76**(5), 823–8.

22 Davies, D. P. (1979). Is inadequate breast-feeding an important cause of failure to thrive? *Lancet*, **1**, 541–2.

23 Hytten, F. E. (1954). Clinical and chemical studies in human lactation VI. The functional capacity of the breast. *British Medical Journal*, **1**, 912–15.

24 Verronen, P. (1982). Breast feeding: Reasons for giving up and transient lactational crises. *Acta Paediatrica Scandinavica*, **71**, 447–50.

25 Hytten, F. E., Yorkston, J. C. and Thompson, A. M. (1958). Difficulties associated with breast-feeding: A study of 106 primiparas. *British Medical Journal*, 1, 310–15.
26 Romito, P. (1988). Mothers' experience of breast feeding. *Journal of Reproductive and Infant Psychology*, 6(2), 89–99.
27 Gray-Donald, K., Kramer, M. S., Munday, S. and Leduc, D. G. (1985). Effect of formula supplementation in the hospital on the duration of breast-feeding: A controlled clinical trial. *Pediatrics*, 75(3), 514–18.

Chapter 10

Childhood asthma: strategies for primary and community health care

Heather Fletcher

Asthma is the most common chronic medical disorder of childhood, affecting approximately 10–15 per cent of children; however, the vast majority of children's asthma can be successfully managed at the primary care level. This chapter considers research carried out during the past decade concerning the prevalence of asthma, influences on its morbidity and mortality, possible outcomes of childhood asthma, and ways in which the best possible management of asthma can be achieved in primary and community care.

Pathology, pathophysiology and drug mechanisms

Asthma is a disorder of the tracheo-bronchial tree in which recurrent obstruction to airflow results in wheeze, cough and shortness of breath; the obstruction is partially or fully reversible. Virtually all children with asthma have increased bronchial responsiveness, which means that their airways narrow too easily and too much in response to a wide range of stimuli (Table 1). Such stimuli or 'trigger factors' can induce both bronchial constriction by contraction of smooth muscle surrounding the bronchial tree, and an inflammatory reaction in the mucosa and submucosal lining of the airways. This reaction includes swelling, accumulation of thick sticky mucus and, in the long term, structural changes which may be irreversible. All these things restrict airflow and breathing needs much more effort. Severe lower airway obstruction causes air to be trapped in the terminal parts of the bronchial tree (the alveoli), which leads to over-inflation of the lungs, impaired gas exchange and eventually the risk of death from hypoxia and ventilatory failure.

Table 1 Some 'trigger factors' for bronchial asthma

Specific	*Non-specific*
Viral infections (most common trigger)	Cold air exposure
Allergens	Exercise
house dust mite	Emotional factors
pollens	
animal danders	
Atmosphere pollutants	
Cigarette smoke	

Three groups of drugs affect various stages of the pathogenetic process. Whereas preventive preparations such as inhaled sodium cromoglycate and inhaled corticosteroids reduce bronchial hyper-responsiveness, bronchodilators achieve direct relaxation of bronchial smooth muscle. Inflammation is reduced both by inhaled and systemic corticosteroids. In all but the mildest cases, it is desirable that the inflammatory component of the condition is treated as well as the smooth muscle constriction. Untreated inflammation renders the airway more hyper-responsive to external trigger factors, and a vicious cycle is established.

The effects of childhood asthma and its outcome

The range of morbidity

The spectrum of childhood asthma is very wide: approximately half of all children with asthma will only have infrequent episodes of cough and mild wheezing; the remainder experience frequent and more severe episodes for many years. About 5–10 per cent of all asthmatics have persistent and often severe airway obstruction; they experience respiratory symptoms on most days of the year and need continuing supervision.

Table 2 lists the problems that can be experienced by asthmatic children, particularly if the asthma is severe or inadequately treated. Nocturnal cough and wheezing may cause sleep disturbance for the entire family. Repeated school absences and restricted performance on the sports field can result in social and academic failure, and loss of self-esteem. A survey of Nottingham school children revealed that 7 per cent of all 5- to 11-year-olds had lost time from school because of wheezing. The median time lost was 7 days per school year but this was thought to be an underestimate.[1] Severe asthmatic attacks are frightening, distressing and dangerous. They may necessitate repeated hospital admissions which are disruptive both to the child and to the family. Finally, poorly controlled severe asthma can result in growth impairment and delayed puberty. It is, therefore, not surprising that emotional and psychological sequelae may complicate childhood asthma.

Table 2 Some effects of childhood asthma

- Disrupted nights and sleep loss
- Repeated school absence
- Exercise restriction
- Hospital admissions
- Life-threatening attacks
- Growth impairment
- Family disruption
- The psychological consequences of chronic childhood illness

Respiratory disease in adulthood

It is commonly thought that childhood asthma is outgrown and, indeed, the majority of children with infrequent and mild asthma do outgrow their symptoms. However, most children with moderate and severe symptoms do not. Furthermore, long-term follow-up studies suggest that some mildly asthmatic children whose symptoms disappear may experience a recurrence of asthma in adulthood.[2] Thus the long-term prognosis for even mild childhood asthma may be less favourable than previously thought and it is possible that so-called 'adult onset' asthma has its origin in childhood. There is also evidence that poor long-term control of symptoms may increase the likelihood of permanent lung damage. A relationship may also exist between childhood asthma, cigarette smoke damage and chronic obstructive lung disease in later life.[3]

Deaths

The condition carries a mortality in children and teenagers of between 0.2 per 100 000 and 1.3 per 100 000 according to age. In England and Wales, 38 children under the age of 15 years died of asthma in 1988 and there were 49 deaths in the 15–19 year age group.[4] Teenage deaths are rising. Preschool children are also vulnerable but death rates appear to be decreasing in this group. This may be a result of more effective modes of drug delivery, earlier hospital admission and improved intensive care facilities. Undoubtedly, most asthma deaths are preventable.[5]

Trends in the prevalence and diagnosis

As most wheezing in children is a manifestation of asthma, studies that have quantified the rates of wheezing illness in a childhood population provide the most accurate prevalence rates.

In the late 1970s, two community surveys on school children in North Tyneside and London revealed prevalence rates of 9.3 and 11.1 per cent, respectively. Only a small proportion of the children surveyed had previously been diagnosed as having asthma, and serious under-recognition and under-treatment of the condition was exposed.[6-8] The publicity given to these findings greatly increased professional awareness of asthma in childhood, and diagnostic rates subsequently improved. A survey of Nottingham school children in 1985 revealed a prevalence rate of 11.5 per cent, half of which were diagnosed. The study was repeated 3 years later and the proportion of children who had been diagnosed rose to 70 per cent.[1,9] A more recent survey in Southampton of 7- and 11-year-old children showed that 80 per cent of the asthmatic children found had already been diagnosed.[10]

There has been continuing controversy as to whether childhood asthma is increasing in Britain.[11] Increases in mortality, hospital admissions and general practice consultations suggest that it may be. However, admission rates are affected by factors such as admitting policy, the willingness of general practitioners (GPs) to refer to hospital and increased parental referral.[12] Likewise, general practice consultation rates are affected by patient expectations and may not necessarily reflect a true rise in asthma. Nevertheless, two recent studies have demonstrated a rise in the prevalence of asthma that cannot be explained by diagnostic or other factors.[13,14]

In summary, increased awareness of unrecognized asthma has led to a significant increase in its diagnosis in the childhood population in the past 10 years. The prevalence of the disease itself is increasing and there is also evidence that other atopic conditions are becoming more common. For example, birth cohort studies demonstrate an increase in reported eczema[15] and there has been a marked increase in general practice consultations for hay fever.[16] The underlying reasons for these trends are unclear. It may be that atopic individuals are becoming exposed to more allergens or that some environmental change is rendering them more susceptible to the effects of allergens. Alternatively, changes may be occurring within the population itself which is increasing its propensity to allergic disease.

The gap between therapeutic developments and their application

During the past 20 years, research into the causes and mechanisms of asthma, and advances in drug therapy and modes of delivery, have revolutionized its management. However, there is still evidence of chronic under-treatment of asthma, despite higher diagnostic rates.[5,10,17,18] This under-treatment can cause frequent and distressing symptoms and even death.

The reasons for this under-treatment and consequent unnecessary morbidity and mortality may involve a number of factors.

The diagnostic 'label'

Previous generations of paediatricians considered that the diagnosis of 'asthma' should be reserved only for severe cases and the term 'bronchitis' was frequently used instead. This meant that children were denied appropriate treatment. In the late 1960s, Australian workers concluded that 'wheezy bronchitis' and asthma were the same thing.[19] While there is continuing debate regarding the use of the 'wheezy bronchitis' label for young children who wheeze in response to viral infections,[20] this distinction is dangerous in practice. A proportion of such children may develop symptoms that warrant aggressive treatment.

Consultation pattern in general practice

Most parents will seek professional help about symptoms that are not normal for their child, and which they consider are potentially serious (see, for example, Chapters 6 and 7, this volume). Parents are very likely to seek medical advice for symptoms such as 'chestiness', 'noisy breathing' or 'chesty cough', often fearing the presence of infection. These may well be signs of asthma. However, a general practice audit of childhood asthma demonstrated that parents made an average of 16 consultations with their children's lower respiratory tract symptoms before the diagnosis of asthma appeared in the practice notes.[21] This study also showed that asthmatic children were brought to the GP more frequently than non-asthmatic children. Short consultations and multiple consultations with different members of a group practice may delay diagnosis: it is quicker to write a prescription for an antibiotic or cough medicine than to take a good history, refer to previous practice records, and provide an explanation and instruction about asthma.

Prescribing practice

Occasionally, bronchodilators may not be prescribed or are prescribed in insufficient quantities because of a lingering fear that inhaled bronchodilators may be dangerous. This may stem from the epidemic of asthma deaths in the 1960s when overuse of inhaled isoprenalin was a suggested but unproven cause. The more selective bronchodilators that have been in use since the early 1970s are thought to be safe. A far more common reason for under-treatment of asthma in general practice is that proper patient assessment is not made, and the need for prophylactic therapy is not considered: far too often there is simple reliance on inhaled bronchodilators. Furthermore, many GPs are reluctant to prescribe corticosteroids for exacerbations. Instead, they prescribe antibiotics that are usually not justified.

Poor compliance and poor patient education

The link between lack of understanding, poor compliance, inadequate self-management and asthma morbidity is obvious. If a child or parent does not understand the prescribed treatment, they are less likely to use it. The drugs most likely to be abandoned are the prophylactic preparations, particularly if the child and parents have neither been taught how to use them, nor why they should be used. Symptoms of asthma are characteristically intermittent and so maintenance drugs may not be considered necessary during asymptomatic periods. Furthermore, compliance may depend on the child's perception of symptoms. Longstanding asthmatics can become remarkably tolerant to impaired lung function: studies comparing the objective degree of airway obstruction and the patient's perception of it have shown that in some cases severe degrees of air flow limitation may be present in the absence of significant subjective symptoms.[22,23] Families may also adapt to chronic symptoms and come to perceive as normal what was once considered abnormal. In adolescents, asthma may have a profound effect on self-image and self-esteem. Symptom tolerance may extend to total denial of the asthma and refusal to take medication. These factors, combined with decreasing parental supervision and lack of effective self-management skills, place the asthmatic adolescent at increased risk of severe attacks and may explain the increased death rates in adolescents and young adults.

The diagnosis and management of asthma in the community

Detection screening programmes

Traditional school entry medical examinations are poor at detecting asthma, but properly designed school screening programmes can be highly success-ful.[24] Questionnaires can be extremely valuable in school-based studies. Providing that a definition of 'wheezing' is given, the single question 'has your child had one or more attacks of wheezing?' can identify up to 96 per cent of asthmatic children.[6] Exercise tests are also a useful screening procedure.[25] However, such programmes can only detect asthma in the age group screened and they miss both pre-school and older children. Thus, while school screening surveys are essential to determine the prevalence of asthma, and may serve as a safety net for asthmatic children who are receiving inadequate care, GPs should be taking more responsibility for the detection and recognition of asthma. Indeed, because the majority of asthmatic children develop their first symptoms before the age of 5 years, detection could be included in pre-school health surveillance.

Making the diagnosis

Usually, the history will suggest the diagnosis, particularly if symptoms are frequent and recurrent. A persistent dry cough is often the only symptom of asthma in some children, who have been shown to have abnormal pulmonary function on exercise tests and to respond to asthma medication.[26]

It is informative to enquire about what factors precipitate the symptoms. In young children, this is invariably upper respiratory tract viral infection, but in severe young asthmatics there may be a history of allergy and exercise-induced wheezing. A personal and/or family history of atopy, such as infantile eczema, can also point to the diagnosis, but its absence should not exclude the diagnosis.

Wheezing is occasionally produced by other conditions such as inhaled foreign body, recurrent aspiration, congenital heart disease, immune deficiency states, bronchiectasis and cystic fibrosis. Although these conditions are very rare in comparison to asthma, they should be considered in the presence of atypical features such as a chronic heavily productive cough, onset in the new born period, association with vomiting, feeding difficulties, failure to thrive, presence of a cardiac murmur or finger clubbing.

Technical investigations such as respiratory function testing, chest X-ray or skin tests are not normally necessary to establish the diagnosis. Between symptomatic episodes, physical examination and peak flow rate are frequently normal. However, where there is uncertainty, a drop in peak flow rate of > 15 per cent at 5 and 10 minutes following a 5-minute period of free running is diagnostic of asthma (free running asthma test: FRAST).[25] Children above the age of 4 years can usually be taught to use peak flow meters.

Continuing assessment

Accurate assessment of every asthmatic child is essential in order to select suitable treatment, to determine the risk of severe attacks and to decide whether specialist referral is necessary. Table 3 lists the questions which should always be asked.

Frequency of symptoms is not invariably related to severity: some may

Table 3 Some key questions to ask in the continuing assessment of children with asthma

---

- How does wheezing affect activity? Can he or she do sports and games? Can he or she run as fast as other children?
- Is he or she missing school? How much absence?
- Is he or she worse at night/early morning?
- Do other things make it worse?
- How often is bronchodilator being used?
- How often do acute attacks occur?
- Any previous hospital admissions?
- Ever been prescribed steroids?
- Is it life-threatening?

---

have frequent mild episodes of wheeze accompanied by minimal consti-
tutional disturbance, whereas others may suffer infrequent but severe
attacks. The provision of a daily record card on which symptoms can be
charted over a period of time is a useful adjunct to the assessment of severity
and response to a particular treatment. Similarly, serial peak flow values are
useful in encouraging self-assessment and management. It is essential to
detect children with marked bronchial lability (wide fluctuations in airway
narrowing), as such children are at considerable risk of severe and dangerous
attacks and require specialist supervision. A detailed description of the child's
condition during their *worst* attack should always be obtained, particularly if
the child is a new patient to the practice. Growth should be regularly
monitored in moderate and severe asthmatics.

Drug therapy

The main aims of drug therapy are: to treat symptomatic episodes early,
thereby relieving acute symptoms and preventing deterioration; to normalize
lung function as far as possible to prevent severe acute episodes and to reduce
the long-term risks of irreversible airflow obstruction and to provide access to
emergency medical treatment.

A recent working party has provided a detailed account of all aspects of the
drug treatment of asthma,[27] here, I simply present an overview. Treatment
should be matched to the age of the child, his or her ability to use inhaler
devices and the severity of the condition. Mild asthmatics (those experiencing
less than one mild to moderate attack per month, or who have minor wheeze
that does not unduly affect activity levels) can be treated with intermittent
bronchodilator. Those experiencing more frequent or more severe attacks
must in addition be prescribed prophylactic inhalers and these should be
taken *continually*. Sodium cromoglycate can be tried initially but more severe
asthmatics frequently require inhaled corticosteroids. Children experiencing
frequent symptoms despite optimal use of prophylaxis need additional
regular bronchodilator or a slow-release bronchodilator to minimize nocturnal wheezing. A small proportion of severe chronic asthmatics who cannot
be controlled on even maximal dosage of bronchodilator and inhaled
corticosteroid may require long-term oral steroid in alternate day doses. This
necessitates careful monitoring and supervision by a paediatrician.

All children and their parents must be taught how to use inhaler devices
properly and their inhaler technique should be checked intermittently. Any
practitioner prescribing them should be able to demonstrate their correct use
and most drug companies provide dummy preparations for practice. It takes
time and patience to ensure that the child can use them competently. There
are practical difficulties in administering inhaled preparations to very young
children. Home nebulizers are particularly useful for administering both
bronchodilator and prophylactic drugs to very young severe asthmatics. Such
children require hospital supervision and meticulous attention to long-term

control. Nebulizers should not be prescribed without explaining their proper use and limitations to parents. By the age of 2½–3 years, spacer devices such as the Nebuhaler and Volumatic can be used. By 5 years, attempts should be made to introduce dry powder inhalers so that the child may be more independent by the time he or she goes to school. The newer breath-activated devices allow effective use at low inspiratory flow rates.

Deteriorating control and acute attacks

There are a number of factors to consider when consulted about worsening asthma: Is the child complying with treatment and how good is his or her inhaler technique? Are there any new provoking factors, e.g. a new pet, cigarette smoke or emotional stress? Is the prescribed treatment adequate? If drug compliance is satisfactory, therapy should be increased. If the response to treatment is still poor, then a short course of oral steroid should be given in addition to existing treatment.

Optimal long-term management should prevent or reduce the occurrence of severe attacks. Nevertheless, children with labile asthma are particularly prone to life-threatening attack. Attacks in young children may be unpredictably severe and even mild asthmatics may occasionally have unexpectedly severe attacks if exposed to a sufficient allergen load. Acute severe attacks require urgent treatment: one survey of asthma deaths revealed that virtually all children who had died following a prolonged attack had either not been treated or had received treatment too late. Medical help had not been sought early enough, or doctors had failed to recognize the severity of the child's condition.[5] Nevertheless, hospital admissions for acute asthma are increasing and the principal reason for this is increased parental referral. GPs are being bypassed in favour of open access to hospital nebulizer treatment and an expectation of hospital admission.[12] While this is a positive indication that more parents are seeking help earlier, it is a sad reflection on the ability of parents and GPs to prevent or deal with acute attacks. We should therefore be encouraging self-reliance by providing the family with the means and confidence to treat acute attacks early and effectively, and providing open hospital access for severe attacks or for those which are not responding to first line therapy. Parents, GPs and hospital consultants should agree to a simple written *crisis plan* (Table 4), which should include advice on the initiation of oral corticosteroids for selected children, a method for delivering high-dose bronchodilator to a breathless child and the indications for immediate transfer to hospital.

The use of aerosol inhalers in conjunction with a large polystyrene coffee cup[28] or a spacer device[29] obviates the need for domiciliary nebulizers and can deliver 1mg of terbutalin or salbutamol. High doses of corticosteroids taken early in an attack reduce its length and severity and prevent dangerous deterioration.[30,31] One recent Canadian study demonstrated a dramatic reduction in hospital admission rates following early intervention with corticosteroids in pre-school children.[32] All moderate and severe asthmatics should initiate such treatment for attacks that fail to respond to high doses of

Table 4 Example of crisis plan for acute attacks

1   BAD ATTACK. USUAL TREATMENT NOT WORKING
    Salbutamol/terbutaline 2.5 mg via nebulizer
 or 10 puffs Salbutamol/terbutaline via spacer. Give one puff every 10 seconds.
 or insert Salbutamol/terbutaline inhaler into base of large polystyrene coffee cup.
    Give 10 puffs at rate of one puff every 10 seconds

2   IF NO RESPONSE
    Start oral prednisolone . . . tablets
      (over 5 years 60 mg; under 5 years 30 mg)
    After 12 hours:
      if wheezing still present, give . . . tablets (2 mg per kg) per day for 2 or 3
      days

3   NOT IMPROVING OR GETTING WORSE
    Consult your doctor urgently˙
 or Take your child directly to hospital˙
    (˙ Delete as applicable)

4   DANGER SIGNS – GO TO HOSPITAL IMMEDIATELY
    Too breathless to talk
    Exhaustion
    Confusion/drowsiness/loss of consciousness
    Chest blown up and hardly moving
    Going blue

bronchodilator. This particularly applies to children on holiday abroad or in remote places, those who use inhaled corticosteroid, those with a history of previous admission and young children. Oral corticosteroids are effective above the age of 18 months but not so in younger infants who require careful medical supervision.[33]

Parents do not generally abuse corticosteroids.[34] Up to 6–8 courses a year can be given without affecting growth and there are data to show that any resulting adrenal suppression is very transient.[35] None the less, a theoretical risk exists in certain children who receive continuous inhaled corticosteroids in combination with four or more courses of oral steroid per year. It is therefore important to document all corticosteroid therapy and in selected cases to consider corticosteroid cover for surgery or major trauma.[36]

Asthma education

Unlike other chronic conditions such as diabetes or cystic fibrosis, we have lagged behind in sharing our knowledge of asthma with our patients. In certain countries, a number of organized asthma education programmes have been established. The best are based on social and behavioural theories that change the role of the child and parents from passive recipients to active participants in the management of asthma. While some subtle beneficial effects have been documented, not all such programmes have been consistently shown to reduce asthma morbidity.[37–39] Education that concentrates on the practical aspects of coping with the condition would appear to be more effective than those focusing on knowledge and understanding. There are a number of broad principles to follow in order to achieve effective asthma education.

Integration

Education cannot be divorced from the medical management of the child, and the professionals involved in his or her long-term care are in the best position to undertake this education. Good rapport and communication between the professionals and the family are essential.

Information

This should be simple and practical. The child and family should have essential core information about what asthma is, how the drugs work, when and how they should be used, and how to avoid allergens (particularly cigarette smoke). Informing and educating are not synonymous however, as information when given alone will not necessarily change motivation or skills in disease management. It is crucial that children and parents are actively taught what to do on a daily basis and how to deal with an acute attack. They should have a clearly written set of instructions. The National Asthma Campaign[40] has introduced two children's asthma cards – one for personal use by parent and child, and the other for schools. Both provide essential information on treatment and emergencies. The Asthma Campaign is also a good resource for written and video educational material.

Beliefs and attitudes

Beliefs and attitudes about asthma are influenced by experience and popular myth and frequently need to be changed in order to achieve good care at home and school. Both child and family must *believe* in their susceptibility to the threatening effects of asthma. Doctors and community nurses should not be diffident in explaining that acute asthma attacks can be dangerous and that poor control both increases the risk of severe attacks and later lung damage. This realistic information does not provoke unnecessary anxiety if the family is provided with a strategy for avoiding severe attacks. Parents and children must be convinced that the treatment works, and therefore it must be acceptable and efficacious. For example, if an aerosol inhaler is prescribed to a child too young to co-ordinate the trigger with inspiration he or she will be deprived of effective treatment and the child and parents will have little confidence in the prescribing doctor. Positive treatment results can be demonstrated to the child by improvement in daily record cards, peak flow rates and exercise tests. Parents are frequently worried about steroids. They need to be reassured that inhaled steroids are totally safe and that occasional short courses of oral steroids have no serious side-effects.,

Timing

Education should be started as early as possible. If educational intervention is provided too late, chronic asthmatics may have become used to their symptoms and feel less motivated to change; this sometimes occurs in families with more than one chronic asthmatic. It is important to remember that only a small percentage of information is absorbed by families at initial consultation. Therefore, this must be checked and reinforced regularly.

Target groups

All children with asthma and their families deserve proper information and education, but certain groups (Table 5) are particularly vulnerable to the life-threatening or chronically disabling effects of the condition. Such children may well be under hospital supervision, but there is the danger that they may fail to attend or become lost to follow-up. Clear arrangements for their supervision should be agreed between the hospital and GP and particular attention devoted to instruction in self-management.

Schools and temporary carers

Child minders, relatives and school teachers should be familiar with the child's asthma and its treatment. Children spend approximately one-third of

Table 5 Children at high risk from asthma

- History of life-threatening episode
- Frequent admissions
- Chronic symptoms requiring long-term oral corticosteroids
- Wide variations in pulmonary function (unstable asthma)
- Severe night-time/early morning symptoms
- Recent discharge from hospital for severe asthma
- Poor self-care/non-compliance
- Severe emotional disturbance
- Manipulative use of asthma
- Family dysfunction

their waking hours in school and an average class may contain 2–3 asthmatic children. Many school teachers do not know how to manage asthma and few know what to do in the case of an acute attack.[41] Parents usually provide some health information to schools but it is the responsibility of the primary and school health services to ensure that accurate written information is available to school staff about asthmatic pupils, their treatment and how to deal with acute attacks. Suitable arrangements should be made for children to use their inhalers in school. School nurses have an important role in educating teaching staff about asthma.

Strategies for the future

The traditional approach to asthma management is clearly inadequate for many families. Brief appointments in busy surgeries and hospital out-patient clinics or frequent emergency consultations and hospital admissions are not conducive to the educational and preventive approaches described in this chapter. These should be integrated with medical management and require time, enthusiasm and good organization.

Specially trained nurses can play a major and developing role in asthma management and education and nurse-run clinics in general practice have been successfully operating in certain parts of the country from as early as 1983.[42–44] The value of such clinics lies in their structured format, consistent approach and in the *time* that the nurse can devote to patient education and support. The National Asthma Campaign runs special training courses for practice nurses and GPs. It has been demonstrated that such clinics are cost-effective in reducing emergency consultations,[45] and are entirely acceptable to patients.

Nurse-run asthma clinics have also been established in certain hospitals' children's out-patient departments. Health education is provided on an individual basis, inhaler technique and peak flow rate are checked, appropriate literature is provided and nebulizers for emergencies and holidays are available on loan. Some of these function on a 'drop in' basis and do not rely on the presence of a doctor,[46] whereas others run in conjunction with normal out-patient clinics. These facilities have been particularly welcomed by parents and have provided a focus for parent support groups. The logical extension is to promote more widespread establishment of these clinics in practice settings to serve the needs of the majority of asthmatic children closer to home.

Another useful procedure is for each health district to establish an 'asthma working group' consisting of a hospital respiratory physician, hospital and community paediatricians, and representatives from health education, nursing, pharmacy and general practice. The group could put particular emphasis on local problems and needs, and could pursue a number of useful objectives. For example, it could develop information systems about local asthma morbidity, e.g. admission rates, consultation rates, detection in schools; it could develop an asthma management strategy for the district; it could set up a training programme for all health professionals involved in the care of children with asthma; and it could promote better services for asthmatic children in the community. All these things would lead to an increase in public knowledge and awareness about the problems of childhood asthma and how to deal with them.

In conclusion, asthma is a common and serious child health problem with unacceptably high morbidity and mortality rates. There is considerable potential for improved management but we will fail to achieve this unless we adopt a positive, committed and organized approach.

References

1 Hill, R. A., Standen, P. J. and Tattersfield, A. E. (1989). Asthma, wheezing and school absence in primary schools. *Archives of Disease in Childhood*, 64, 246–51.
2 Kelly, W. J. W., Hudson, I., Phelan, P. D., Pain, M. C. F. and Olinsky, A. (1987). Childhood asthma in adult life: A further study at 28 years of age. *British Medical Journal*, 294, 1059–62.
3 Pearlman, D. S. (1984). Bronchial asthma: A perspective from childhood to adulthood. *American Journal of Diseases in Childhood*, 138, 459–66.
4 Office of Population Censuses and Surveys: Medical Statistics Unit (personal communication).
5 Fletcher, H. J., Ibrahim, S. A. and Speight, A. N. P. (1990). Survey of asthma deaths in the Northern Region 1970–1985. *Archives of Disease in Childhood*, 65, 163–7.
6 Lee, D. A., Winslow, N. R., Speight, A. N. P. and Hey, E. N. (1983). Prevalence and spectrum of asthma in childhood. *British Medical Journal*, 286, 1256–8.
7 Anderson, H. R., Bailey, P. A., Cooper, J. S., Palmer, S. C. and West, S. (1983). Morbidity and school absence caused by asthma and wheezing illness. *Archives of Disease in Childhood*, 58, 777–84.
8 Speight, A. N. P., Lee, D. A. and Hey, E. N. (1983). Underdiagnosis and undertreatment of asthma in childhood. *British Medical Journal*, 286, 1253–6.
9 Hill, R., Williams, J., Tattersfield, A. and Britton, J. (1989). Change in the use of asthma as a diagnostic label for wheezing illness in school children. *British Medical Journal*, 299, 898.
10 Clifford, R. D., Radford, M., Howell, J. B. and Holgate, J. T. (1989). Prevalence of respiratory symptoms among 7 and 11 year old school children and association with asthma. *Archives of Disease in Childhood*, 64, 1118–25.
11 Anderson, H. R. (1989). Is the prevalence of asthma changing? *Archives of Disease in Childhood*, 64, 172–5.
12 Storr, J., Barrell, E. and Lenney, W. (1988). Rising asthma admissions and self referral. *Archives of Disease in Childhood*, 63, 774–9.
13 Burr, M. L., Butland, B. K., King, S. and Vaughan-Williams, E. (1989). Changes in asthma prevalence: Two surveys 15 years apart. *Archives of Disease in Childhood*, 64, 1452–6.
14 Burney, P. G. J., Chinn, S. and Rona, R. J. (1990). Has the prevalence of asthma increased in children?: Evidence from the national study of health and growth 1973–86. *British Medical Journal*, 300, 1306–10.

15 Taylor, B., Wadsworth, J., Wadsworth, M. and Peckham, C. (1984). Changes in the prevalence of reported eczema since the 1939–45 war. *Lancet*, ii, 1255–7.

16 Fleming, D. M. and Crombie, D. L. (1987). Prevalence of asthma and hay fever in England and Wales. *British Medical Journal*, 294, 279–83.

17 Zeiden, S., Ali, H., Danskin, M. J. and Hey, E. N. (1988). The temporal pattern and natural history of asthma in childhood. Abstract of the British Paediatric Association Annual General Meeting.

18 Conway, S. P. and Littlewood, J. M. (1985). Admission to hospital with asthma. *Archives of Disease in Childhood*, 60, 636–9.

19 Williams, H. E. and McNicol, K. N. (1969). Prevalence, natural history and relationship of wheezy bronchitis and asthma in children: An epidemiological study. *British Medical Journal*, 4, 321–5.

20 Wilson, N. M. (1989). Wheezy bronchitis revisited. *Archives of Disease in Childhood*, 64, 1194–9.

21 Levy, M. and Bell, L. (1984). General practice audit of asthma in childhood. *British Medical Journal*, 289, 1115–16.

22 Rubinfield, A. R. and Pain, M. C. F. (1976). Perception of asthma. *Lancet*, i, 882–4.

23 Burdon, G. W., Juniper, E. F., Killain, K. J., Hargreave, F. E. and Campbell, E. J. M. (1982). The perception of breathlessness in asthma. *American Review of Respiratory Disease*, 126, 825–8.

24 Colver, A. F. (1984). Community campaign against asthma. *Archives of Disease in Childhood*, 59, 449–52.

25 Tsanakas, J. N., Milner, R. D. G., Bannister, O. M. and Boon, A. W. (1988). Free running asthma screening test. *Archives of Disease in Childhood*, 63, 261–5.

26 Konig, P. (1981). Hidden asthma in childhood. *American Journal of Disease in Childhood*, 135, 1053–5.

27 Warner, J. O., Gotz, M., Landau, L. I., Levison, H., Milner, A. D., Pederson, S. and Silverman, M. (1989). Management of asthma: A consensus statement. *Archives of Disease in Childhood*, 64, 1065–79.

28 Henry, R. L., Milner, A. D. and Davis, J. G. (1989). Simple drug delivery system for use by young asthmatics. *British Medical Journal*, 286, 20–1.

29 Freelander, M. and Van 'Asperen, P. P. (1984). Nebuhaler versus Nebuliser in children with acute asthma. *British Medical Journal*, 288, 1873–4.

30 Deshpande, A. and McKenzie, S. A. (1986). Short course of steroids in home treatment of children with acute asthma. *British Medical Journal*, 293, 169–71.

31 Storr, J., Barry, W., Barrell, E. and Lenny, W. (1987). Effect of a single oral dose of prednisolone in acute childhood asthma. *Lancet*, i, 879–82.

32 Brunette, M. G., Lands, L. and Thibodear, L. P. (1988). Childhood asthma: Prevention of attacks with short term corticosteroid treatment of upper respiratory tract infection. *Pediatrics*, 81, 624–9.

33 Webb, M. S. C., Henry, R. L. and Milner, A. D. (1986). Oral corticosteroids for wheezing attacks under 18 months. *Archives of Disease in Childhood*, 61, 15–19.

34 Hosker, H. (1987). The use of home administered short courses of corticosteroid in childhood asthma. Paper presented at the European Paediatric Respiratory Society, Helsinki.

35 Zora, J. A., Zimmerman, D., Earey, T. L., O'Connel, E. J. and Yunginger, J. W. (1986). Hypothalamic-pituitary-adrenal axis suppression after short term high dose glucocorticoid therapy in children with asthma. *Journal of Allergy and Cinical Immunology*, 77, 9–13.

36 Dolan, L. M., Kersarwala, H. H., Holroyde, J. C. and Fischer, T. J. (1987). Short term, high dose, systemic steroids in children with asthma: The effect on the hypothalamic-pituitary-adrenal axis. *Journal of Allergy and Clinical Immunology*, 80, 81–7.
37 Howland, J., Bauchner, H. and Adair, R. (1988). The impact of paediatric asthma education on morbidity: Assessing the evidence. *Chest*, 94, 964–9.
38 Mitchell, E. A., Ferguson, V. and Norwood, M. (1986). Asthma education by community child health nurses. *Archives of Disease in Childhood*, 61, 1184–9.
39 Wilson Pessano, S. R. and Mellins, R. B. (1987). Workshop on asthma self management: Summary of workshop discussion. *Journal of Allergy and Clinical Immunology*, 80, 4, 489–91.
40 The National Asthma Campaign, 300 Upper St, London N1 2XX, UK.
41 Reynolds, M. A., Ayward, P. and Heaf, D. P. (1988). How much do school teachers know about asthma? *Paediatric Review Community*, 2, 173–80.
42 Barnes, G. (1988). Asthma: Latest developments in care. *The Professional Nurse*, June, 364–8.
43 Charlton, I. (1989). Asthma clinics: Setting up. *Practitioner*, 233, 1359–62.
44 Charlton, I. (1989). Asthma clinics: How to run one. *Practitioner*, 233, 1440–45.
45 Charlton, I. (1989). Asthma clinics: Audit. *Practitioner*, 233, 1522–3.
46 Wooler, E. (1989). The provision of a 'drop in' clinic for the asthmatic child. *Respiratory Disease in Practice*, 6, 8–10.

Chapter 11

Child sexual abuse and the trials of motherhood

Jenny Kitzinger

The child who has been sexually assaulted feels confused, dirty and ashamed. When her attacker is her own father (or stepfather, uncle or grandfather), she feels particularly betrayed and unloved because she has been exploited by someone who was supposed to care for her.[1] The reactions of those around her – friends, relatives and professionals – are important in helping her to cope with what has happened. Above all, her mother plays a crucial role in comforting and reassuring the child, freeing her from guilt and helping to restore her self-confidence.[2,3] It is the mother–child relationship that forms the focus of this chapter. Drawing on interviews with six women whose daughters were abused and 39 women who were themselves abused I ask: How do mothers and children feel after abuse is discovered? What notions of 'good' or 'bad' mothering inform intervention? How can health care professionals support the mother and thus also the child?[2]

Discovering abuse

When a woman first learns that her child has been abused her initial reaction is often one of horror and disbelief. There is rarely incontrovertible medical evidence and the abuser usually vehemently protests his innocence while the child's own statements may be tentative or veiled. One child left a poem in her room describing abuse, another showed her mother an article in a women's magazine, a third simply told her mother that her daddy 'tasted funny'. The mother may not know what to believe and may reject her own suspicions as crazy. Kathy first realized something was wrong when she was woken up one night by her 9-year-old daughter's sobs:

> I found that my husband must have heard her first because he'd got up and was out of bed, he had obviously gone to see her. I got up and he said that she was OK and told me to go back to bed. But she was obviously still crying so I didn't. At which point he went back to bed and she told me that she had had a dream that a man had come into her bedroom and touched her. She said it was a dream but she also was more upset than if it had been a dream.

Some 'gut reaction' told Kathy to take what Rose was saying very seriously and she took her to see a doctor. The first general practitioner (GP) she saw, however, was not very helpful.

> He didn't know how to cope with it all really, he said it probably *was* a dream. . . . He said, children did make things up occasionally and I shouldn't worry too much about it.

It was only because of Kathy's persistence (she went back to see another GP) and the constant reassurance she gave to her daughter that Rose was able to admit that in fact Kathy's husband (Rose's stepfather) had been sexually assaulting her.

Mother-blaming

Once a woman has overcome her child's, and her own, fears about confronting the abuse (and possible professional resistance), she may be faced with overwhelming guilt and a devastating sense of failure. Unfortunately, intervention by doctors, friends, and health and community workers can reinforce such feelings. One of the most destructive assumptions about mothers of abused children is that they are 'collusive', 'incompetent' or 'neglectful'. The mother's dereliction of duty is apparently proved by the fact that harm has come to her child. The questions I am most commonly asked when talking about incest to both lay and professional groups are: 'How could the mother not have known?' and 'Why didn't she do anything?'

Often these are the questions with which mothers themselves struggle. They wonder why they were not suspicious when their partners volunteered to bathe the children or read them bedtime stories, or kept getting out of bed ostensibly to go to the toilet. In retrospect, they now realize that these were all opportunities for abuse. Women who went out to work felt guilty for not being available to their children; those who stayed at home felt guilty that, despite being at home, they did not notice what was going on – '. . . it wasn't as if I wasn't around – I was there for them. I should have seen what was happening. I was incompetent as a mother.' They felt that they lacked a 'true' mother's intuition about their child's well-being. When Amy discovered that the (male) babysitter had abused her 3-year-old daughter, she felt particularly bad because she herself had been abused as a child: 'I felt "damn, I thought I'd be safe from that. Me going through it, I should have known." I felt very like I weren't good enough again. I was really down.'

Not only are women made to feel guilty for not knowing about the abuse but they are held responsible for 'allowing' it to happen in the first place. If a mother neglects to chaperon her children 24 hours a day, even when in the company of their own father, this may be used to obscure or mitigate the abuser's guilt. As one lawyer, defending a man accused of sexually abusing his daughter, declared: 'This woman repeatedly went to the grocery store leaving this child alone with her father.'[4] The abuser himself often tries to transfer responsibility onto the woman:

> He said I was to blame for this. If I were a wise and knowledgeable mother, my children would have been armed, and he couldn't have done what he did because they would have been protected.[5]

The mother is thus portrayed as culpably negligent and sometimes she is even identified as the root cause of the abuse. Some mothers are labelled 'incest carriers'; it is argued that because of their own childhood abuse they grow up to choose men who will abuse their children.[6] Sexual abuse is described rather like a disease (such as haemophilia), carried by females but activated primarily in males. Alternatively, mothers are identified as the cause of sexual violence because they have 'largely opted out of normal wifely and maternal functions'[7] or a woman may be accused of '. . . renting out her daughter in return for neglecting to make any attempt to create a warm and loving relationship for him or her family'.[8]

Assumptions about women's responsibility for protecting children and taking care of men (including men's sexual needs) have a direct impact on the help offered to women whose children have been abused. Rather than aiming to restore women's self-esteem and focusing on their strengths and mothering skills, much lay and professional treatment of mothers serves to disempower them. Indeed, some intervention, drawing on the family dysfunction model, explicitly encourages mothers to recognize their own complicity and realize that nothing will be solved by 'scapegoating' the abusers and allying themselves with their abused offspring. One therapist, for example, states:

> The mother's first reaction is often to want to leave. This will be expressed in the form of a wish for immediate divorce, or she may attempt to collude [sic] with her daughter against the father.

With the appropriate help, however,

> the wife's initial disappointment and hatred of her husband soon give way to the depressing realisation that she has failed, not only as a good mother, but also as a partner.[9]

Mothers, then, should be encouraged to admit that they are implicated in the abuse and we are warned that 'when the mother's role in the incest becomes a more central issue, the therapist has to be prepared for serious suicidal attempts on the part of the mother'.[10] A woman's self-confidence is undermined (to the point of triggering suicide attempts) at the time she most needs support. Not surprisingly, some of the mothers I interviewed described becoming increasingly depressed, defensive and guilt-ridden during the course of professional intervention. They learn to condemn themselves for being too sexually passive or too sexually demanding, for being too submissive (and thus providing a poor role model for their daughter) or too strong (and thus driving their husbands to exercise power over weaker members of the family). In fact, whatever a woman does she can find some fault in her behaviour: 'I felt guilty about it because maybe something I did caused it to happen,' says one woman; 'I felt ashamed about it because of other people's reactions and because it had made me feel dirty. I felt "did I do something that caused it? Was I not a good enough wife, was I too dominant?".' Similarly, another woman recites a litany of self-accusations:

> And I'd stayed with him so long, for the sake of the children. And maybe he abused her because I wasn't prepared, at that point, to have sex with him, except involuntarily. . . . And when she was nine, I knew she didn't want to go to visit her father but I made her go because I had this idea that the children *ought* to see their father.

In retrospect, this woman feels guilty even for those attempts to be a 'good mother': struggling to preserve her marriage for so long and, after divorce, encouraging the children to maintain a relationship with their father.

'She's punishing me': the ongoing mother–child relationship

At the same time as having her confidence undermined, a woman is faced with the most frightening and demanding time of her relationship with her child. Many mothers are haunted by the destructive media spectre of the abuse victim as a 'walking time-bomb' who is 'scarred for life'. They worry that their child will never be 'normal' or 'happy' and their fears are exacerbated if the child begins to display after-effects such as night terrors, self-mutilation, sexualized behaviour, refusal to eat or to go to school, depression and violence (sometimes aimed at the mother, younger children or animals). The child may recoil from hugs or she may become very clingy and dependent and start thumb-sucking or bed-wetting. Having been betrayed and abused by one parent she fears being rejected or abandoned by the other ('I though that if my mother knew she would think I was dirty and would never cuddle me every again'). The child is desperate for reassurance and demands unconditional love and acceptance.

While continually testing out her mother's love the abused child may also express a great deal of anger against her. This is especially true if she thinks that her mother was aware of, and condoned, the abuse all along. Children are often convinced that their mothers did know, or should have known, what was happening. After all, mothers have the uncanny ability to detect who ate that last piece of chocolate cake and when an illness is being faked in an attempt to avoid going to school; therefore, how could mummy *not* know what daddy was doing? In addition, some abusers deliberately alienate the victimized child from the rest of the family and protect themselves by ensuring that the child has a reputation for lying:

> He was living within a knife edge of me telling someone. He then became very vicious, he would say things to my brother and sister like 'Don't you ever believe anything that child says, she's illegitimate, the lowest of the low.' He completely marginalised me in the family and that includes my mother.

If the child is already viewed as 'bad', then she may be seen as 'out to make trouble', and if the abuser has convinced the child that her mother is 'bad', the child may be equally mistrustful in return. Such estrangement between mother and child is often viewed as a 'pre-condition' for abuse, whereas it might more properly be seen as a consequence. The child may also hold the mother responsible for what happens *after* disclosure. She will be angry if her mother fails to seek help and stays with the abuser (which usually means that the abuse continues); she may, however, also feel betrayed if her mother reports the abuse, leaves the abuser and the child is forced to repeat her story to a host of strangers (if the abuser has treated the child as his 'little princess' and cast the mother as the 'wicked witch' the child may feel great loyalty to her father despite the abuse).

Conflict between mother and child can escalate during this period: 'She's punishing me, every day she punishes me. She treats me like dirt. She's become a hateful, terrified little monster', said one woman. At the same time, discovering the abuse can leave the woman feeling very isolated and totally responsible for her child: 'Their father doing that to them really brought it home to me – these kids are my responsibility and mine alone. I can't trust them to anyone else. It's me and them, and no one else.'

'It was wonderful to have someone to turn to': the role of professionals

Community health practitioners have a vital role in combating this isolation and helping to alleviate what can become a claustrophobic and fraught relationship riddled with guilt and anger on both sides. First, workers may be able to provide a listening ear to the child (especially the older child) if she wishes to talk to a sympathetic outsider who is not directly involved. Secondly, they can draw on their professional power and expertise to provide women with a great deal of practical information and back-up (ranging from helping to remove the abuser from the home through to ideas about how the child might be feeling). Careful discussion can help the mother to understand her child's behaviour as well as clarifying her own reactions.

However, intervention that starts from the presumption of maternal failure can be undermining instead of supportive. Once it is known that child sexual abuse has occurred within the family, the mother's conduct comes under close scrutiny and she can be subject to a barrage of advice from a variety of well-meaning professionals. Often, the traditional white, middle-class model of family life promoted by these professionals takes little account of the constraints of either time or money available to the mother and fails to acknowledge her existing mothering skills. State intervention can be profoundly threatening and black or working-class mothers are often pre-judged by the system. As one working-class woman comments: 'To someone like me, social workers are something you keep away from. I thought they'd take the kids away from me and it would be someone else telling me I'm not good enough.'

Even white, middle-class mothers may find that their own ways of relating to their children are dismissed and they are expected to adopt an alien style of mothering. For example, one influential theory states that incest results from a failure to maintain intergenerational boundaries; some practitioners thus urge women to restore traditional family divisions by adopting a firm and protecting mothering style and taking responsibility for all decisions. Such an approach suits some women and children but unwavering adherence to this theory can lead workers to disregard the strengths of the existing mother–child alliance. Evelyn and her teenage daughter have striven to create an egalitarian, honest and mutually respectful relationship, but Evelyn's social worker persists in promoting a different model of how they should relate. She tells Evelyn that she is 'colluding' with the abuser by failing to confront him (even though Evelyn has not done so out of respect for her daughter's own wishes). Evelyn feels she is constantly in conflict with her social workers over what a family should be like: 'I find this social worker very disabling' she says, '. . . when I'm with her she seems so definite and seems to know what she is talking about'. Her daughter, Sarah, is equally uncomfortable with the social worker's attitudes at times. On one occasion, for example, the social worker told Evelyn that she must take responsibility for keeping her daughter safe and gave the example of making sure Sarah was on the pill. It was Sarah who challenged the social worker's assumptions and declared that her choice of contraception was her responsibility, *not* her mother's.

Along with respecting the woman's knowledge of her own daughter it is also vital that practitioners recognize her feelings as a woman in her own right. Unfortunately, the concern of professionals (and the woman herself) for the 'best interests of the child' often leads them to forget that discovering that a loved and trusted man is a child abuser is a trauma for the mother as well as the victim. 'What he had done was so awful that I just wanted to wash it away. It made me feel dirty. It made me feel tainted to be his wife.' The mother's feelings are, in fact, very similar to those of an actual rape victim.[11] Her faith in her own judgement is torn apart, her trust in other people destroyed, her whole life is thrown into turmoil. Women talk of being trapped in some kind of horrific time warp: 'It is a horrible feeling of numbness as though the world has stopped still and mentally you can't function backwards or forwards';[12] 'I couldn't look forward at all and I was blocking out a lot of the past, just cut both off.'

Instead of allowing mothers space to talk, some practitioners simply advise women to restrain any display of emotions in front of their children. From the children's point of view this may be good advice – children often fear that knowledge of the abuse will destroy their mothers, they become very watchful and wary and feel responsible for all the pain and grief experienced by other members of the family. If the mother seems overwhelmed by horror, then the child may well retract the accusations. On the other hand, maintaining a reserved and cautious response can be difficult for the mother may be misunderstood by the child. One woman, whose GP gave her a supply of valium and urged her to carry on as normally as possible, described how her daughter later turned on her saying her lack of emotional response meant she must have known all along and that her calm insistence on carrying on as if nothing had happened denied the impact of the abuse on the whole family.

Whether or not it is appropriate to share their feelings with their children, women do need some acknowledgement of their own anger, disgust, shame and confusion. However, they may be wary of confiding in professionals, especially if the workers who offer help are the same workers who might be called upon to give evidence in care proceedings. Women feel obliged to keep up a positive front, proving that they are stable and competent mothers – 'coping' is, after all, the essential ingredient of adequate mothering and not being able to cope is a damning indictment which could be the first step in losing custody of their children.[13] Women may also avoid acknowledging their own feelings for fear of being overwhelmed by them and some deliberately neglect their own well-being: 'You feel that you don't deserve to have any care, worry about yourself, you don't deserve any protection because you shouldn't have let it happen.'

The self-sacrificing mother: Kathy's (and Rose's) story

Kathy, in many ways, represents 'The Ideal Mother'. She is passionately committed to her children and, from the moment she suspected abuse, acted to protect them. Describing the first night when her daughter told her of the 'dream' in which she had been abused, Kathy says:

> I remember lying in bed with her and just holding her until she went off to sleep and trying to ease something from her and at the same time as I was trying to ease it from her it was getting worse and worse for me. It was horrible, it was really like a whole night of nightmares and when daylight came it wouldn't have happened. But it didn't go away.

The next morning she made her husband leave the house. The subsequent 2 years were spent coping with practical arrangements and struggling to keep her job as well as caring for a very disturbed 9-year-old daughter and the indirect impact on her younger sons. At the same time, she had to deal with continual phone calls from her husband demanding that she help him (on one occasion he turned up on her doorstep having taken an overdose and it was Kathy who had to take him to hospital). She described these 2 years in terms of 'getting by' and 'living minute by minute'.

At the beginning, Rose was very disturbed and unhappy, she had great outbursts of rage where she became violent and lost all control. For example, on one occasion, Rose knocked Kathy back off a bed and over a chair:

> I lay on the floor and I thought 'You can't have broken your back, if you've broken your back you can't get up off this floor and cope with her in five minutes time', so I said 'right, you haven't broken your back, get up'. Ooh, and was I bruised and sore for days! But I remember lying on the floor and thinking 'don't be so stupid you cannot break your back, because if you do what is going to happen?' And that is how I just lived.

During this time, Kathy was 'a tower of strength'. However, after 2 years of struggling from crisis to crisis, she became severely, and in her view 'inexplicably' depressed:

> I'd sorted everything out and that was going to be the end of it. And nobody needed me to cope any more. . . . I'd sorted out her school, I'd moved house, I'd got the divorce. . . . I kept asking myself 'why are you feeling like this, you've sorted everything out, everything is fine'. But I just felt so depressed but I didn't know why. There was no reason for it.

Her doctor had told her that it could take up to 2 years to get over what had happened:

> . . . so I had two months to go before the two years were up. Something in my head told me that I should be getting over it. But I knew I wasn't. And I couldn't tell anybody, I had to be alright superficially to everybody. . . . I started to get up every morning with that dead weight across my shoulders. I just didn't know what to do, I didn't know how to feel any better. I was just dragging myself about. One day I went home and I had an old bottle of anti-depressants there that the doctor had given me at the beginning and I got them out of the cupboard and took them. Then I lay down on the settee. I just wanted to escape, I just wanted to stop the bad feeling.

Kathy was rushed to hospital by an alert psychiatric social worker who was so concerned about her that he called round at her house that afternoon. It was only after this that Kathy (and those around her) realized that she needed care and attention in her own right. As Kathy herself put it, she had to have support, if only for the sake of the children:

> I got to the point where I nearly killed myself and left my children. You

can't get further than that. So I knew that I had got to heal myself to be any good, to bring them up for the rest of their childhood.

Conclusion

Discussion of the role of mothers in cases of child sexual abuse repeatedly conjures up the image of the 'good', 'true' or 'real' (as opposed to the 'bad', 'inadequate' or 'unnatural') mother. Health care professionals, child sexual abuse 'experts' and the women themselves often draw on a notion of motherhood as a selfless state, an all-seeing, all-nurturing, all-protective and all-powerful role. This ideal ignores the material realities of women's lives and places an insupportable burden on mothers – charging them with total responsibility for their offspring's physical, mental and emotional well-being. It is not surprising that so many women judge themselves, and are judged by others (including their children), to have failed.

Community health practitioners can provide a vital support system for women and children, breaking through the isolation of the family; however, often intervention instead serves as a form of policing. Women's own ways of mothering are condemned, they are cross-questioned about their behaviour (with loaded queries such as 'Were you having sex with your husband during this time?'); they are labelled 'chaotic', 'collusive' or 'neglectful' and vilified for failing to live up to the dominant culture's maternal and wifely ideal. Alternatively, a woman may find herself on the pedestal reserved for 'good' mothers ('She's wonderful, I don't know how she copes') – a pedestal which traps her in a self-destructive, self-sacrificing role with no space to consider her own needs and human limitations.

We need to question the underlying social construction of maternal protection (and the interdependent construction of childhood vulnerability),[14] recognize the difficulties women face and refuse to perpetuate the unrealistic demands placed upon them to carry on coping regardless. This means ensuring that all community health workers build up some knowledge about the impact of abuse on mothers as well as children and that they are able to give women access to legal, financial and practical help. By signalling concern for, and a commitment to, the woman and consistently treating her with care and respect, workers can become a resource for her instead of part of the system used against her. By challenging stereotypical notions of good and bad mothering, workers can help to reinforce a strong mother–child relationship and offer advocacy instead of criticism, and support instead of condemnation.

Notes and references

1 Because my own work has been around the abuse of girls and women and because of the gender politics of sexual violence (most perpetrators are male, most victims

female), I refer to the child as 'she' throughout. Most of the issues addressed in this chapter are, however, also relevant to women who have sons.

2 Summit, R. (1983). The child sexual abuse accommodation syndrome. *Child Abuse and Neglect*, 7, 177–93.

3 Hildebrand, J. and Forbes, C. (1987). Group work with mothers whose children have been sexually abused. *British Journal of Social Work*, 17, 285–304.

4 MacFarlane, K. (1988). Current issues in child sexual abuse. Talk given at *Intervening in Child Sexual Abuse*, Glasgow.

5 Johnson, J. (1985). Ethnographic study of mothers in father–daughter incest families. PhD thesis, University of Pennsylvania.

X 6 Hancock, M. and Burton Mains, B. (1987). *Child Sexual Abuse: A Hope for Healing*. Illinois, Harold Shaw.

7 Report of the Howard League Working Party (1985). *Unlawful Sex*. London, Waterloo Publications.

8 Pizzey, E. and Dunne, M. (1980). Sexual abuse within the family. *New Society*, 13 November, 312–14.

X 9 Furniss, T. (1983). Family process in the treatment of intrafamilial child sexual abuse. *Journal of Family Therapy*, 5, 263–78.

10 Furniss, T. (1983). Op. cit., p. 276.

11 De Jong, A. (1988). Maternal responses to the sexual abuse of their children. *Pediatrics*, 8(1), 14–21.

12 Hooper, C.-A. (1987). Getting him off the hook: The theory and practice of mother blaming in child sexual abuse. *Trouble and Strife*, 12, 20–25.

13 Graham, H. (1982). Coping: Or how mothers are seen and not heard. In Friedman, S. and Sarah, E. (eds), *On The Problem of Men: Two Feminist Conferences*. London, Women's Press.

14 Kitzinger, J. (1990). Who are you kidding? Children, power and the struggle against sexual abuse. In James, A. and Prout, A. (eds), *Constructing and Reconstructing Childhood*. London, Falmer Press.

Chapter 12

Children with HIV infection: their care in the community

Jacqueline Mok

The Acquired Immunodeficiency Syndrome (AIDS) was first recognized in young homosexual men in the early 1980s, when unusual infections and cancers were seen. The Human Immunodeficiency Virus (HIV) was identified as the infectious agent and the modes of transmission documented as: unprotected homosexual and heterosexual sexual intercourse; the receipt of infected blood and blood products (including the sharing of contaminated needles and syringes) and from an infected woman to her child before birth. With the routine screening of donors, the numbers of individuals infected by blood and blood products should be on the decline. Changes in sexual practice in the male homosexual community have also resulted in decreasing numbers of gay men acquiring new infection. Heterosexual transmission remains the most difficult route to eradicate, and HIV is now known to be infecting increasing numbers of women, with obvious consequences for children born to infected women.

In Edinburgh, studies of injecting drug misusers (IDM's) revealed that the first HIV seropositive tests were recorded in late 1983, with subsequent seroprevalence rates reported to vary from 38 to 54 per cent.[1-3] These HIV positive reports came mainly from the Lothian region, where an estimated 2000 drug misusers are registered, one-third of whom are young, sexually active women. Unlike many centres in the UK where HIV has infected the male homosexual population, the problems seen in Edinburgh have involved heterosexual transmission from men to women and women to men, as well as vertical transmission from mother to child.

Clinical spectrum of HIV infection in children

Little is known about the rates of HIV transmission from mother to child, or about the natural history of perinatally acquired HIV disease, but on-going prospective studies of HIV-infected children have revealed that children present with an extremely wide variety of clinical signs and symptoms: failure to thrive, recurrent respiratory infections, chronic diarrhoea, unexplained fever, generalized lymphadenopathy and hepatosplenomegaly. The general-ized nature of this range of symptoms and signs means that general practitioners (GPs) or health visitors will probably be the first professionals to be presented with these problems.

There is a bimodal age distribution of children manifesting symptoms and signs of HIV disease. Those who present within the first year of life do so with rapidly progressive disease affecting either the lung (pneumocystis carinii pneumonia) or the central nervous system (encephalopathy), and their mortality is high. Children with recurrent bacterial infections, lymphocytic interstitial pneumonitis (LIP), generalized lymphadenopathy or nephropathy tend to survive longer. If the child's gastrointestinal system is affected, malnutrition and severe wasting are severe problems. Anaemia is also seen, along with bleeding disorders when the platelet count is low. It is clear that HIV can affect any organ, either directly or indirectly.

However, some infected children remain completely healthy, or may have only minor common childhood complaints for several years. These children will obviously remain undetected until medical advice is sought for symptoms relating to a defective immune system.

Diagnosis of HIV infection in children

Diagnosis of HIV infection in children is based on the suspicion of clinical findings together with epidemiological risk factors in the child or mother (primarily injecting drug misuse), and confirmed by laboratory tests. In adults, a positive HIV antibody test is a reliable and sensitive indicator of infection. However, the fact that HIV antibodies are transferred passively from mother to baby pre-natally means that antibody testing is not a useful diagnostic tool in infants under the age of 18 months. While a positive antibody test over this age implies HIV infection, a negative test does not necessarily exclude infection as some infected children may not mount an antibody response at all, while others may show a delayed response after several years. The time to seroconversion in children is unknown. Where available, virus culture or antigen tests are useful as diagnostic tools when antibody results are confusing, although the lack of sensitivity of the tests means that negative results do not rule out the possibility of infection either. Other helpful laboratory tests include lymphocyte subsets (especially the CD4 count), immunoglobulin levels and platelet counts.

Confidentiality and HIV testing

Confidentiality and the role of HIV testing are important issues when dealing with children who might be infected with HIV and their families, or potential foster or adoptive families. As 80 per cent of children infected with HIV have been infected by vertical transmission, and because a positive HIV test in a child implies the mother is also infected, good clinical practice would dictate that parental consent for testing should be obtained whenever possible. None the less, the British Medical Association has stated that children can be tested without parental consent if it is essential to the child's care that the HIV status were known.

HIV testing is not warranted for children who are placed for foster care because evidence against the casual transmission of the virus is mounting, and day-to-day activities in foster families carry no risk of transmission. Many injecting drug users have also been infected with the hepatitis B virus, which can be transmitted from mother to child and is much more infectious than HIV. It may be more pertinent to test the child's hepatitis B status, or to ensure that foster families are protected against hepatitis B by vaccination.

The issue is more complicated concerning adoption. Adoption agencies are required to give medical information about children to prospective adopters supposedly to promote the welfare of the child placed for adoption. A woman placing her child for adoption should be counselled about her and her partner's lifestyle to identify any risk activities for HIV infection, and requested to have tests for HIV infection. If permission is refused, or if the mother is not available, the agency should outline to the adoptive parents the possible risks of HIV infection and what this might mean to a child. Prospective adopters need a good understanding that an antibody test may not be useful in a young infant and should be given an opportunity for full discussions with a medical adviser knowledgeable in these issues. Testing of the child could occur in future, at the request of the adoptive parents, upon granting of the adoption order. Adoption agencies should be wary of prospective adopters who seek an absolute guarantee that the child is free from HIV infection. In areas of high HIV prevalence, that guarantee can never be given, and the suitability of the prospective adopters must be questioned.

Medical management of infected children

Most children with HIV infection come from multiple-deprived families, who have many social, family, financial and health problems, and usually a problem with injecting drug misuse. In addition, the child's mother is usually infected and may manifest various stages of the disease at the same time that her child is ill. Thus professional and voluntary agencies face complex challenges in dealing with children with HIV infection. Therapeutic programmes are doomed to failure if family, social and financial difficulties are not recognized;

or if cooperation between medical, nursing, social work and voluntary staff is not achieved. Community health workers are particularly important in supporting families to care for children with HIV disease at home.

A study comparing pregnancy outcomes for HIV positive compared to HIV negative women in Edinburgh[4] found no differences between the two groups for a number of adverse outcomes: preterm delivery, intrauterine growth retardation, or low birth weight. However, the whole group was characterized as deprived, and with lifestyles which could have adversely affected the pregnancy outcome, and had twice the rate of prematurity and intrauterine growth retardation compared to rates for Edinburgh as a whole, and four times as many low birthweight babies.

Good nutrition is vital for HIV-infected children to maintain optimal growth. Advice from a paediatric dietitian is essential, although low-income families may find it difficult to comply with dietetic advice. Supplementary benefits may be available to some families, and they should be made aware of these benefits. HIV disease of the gastrointestinal tract, or infectious complications might necessitate parenteral feeding. But once this has been established in hospital, some families can cope with the care of an indwelling catheter at home, with the help and support of community nurses.

Children with recurrent bacterial infections may benefit from regular infusions of gammaglobulin,[5] or the use of long-term broad-spectrum antibiotics. Health professionals should encourage parents to seek medical advice if common infections persist despite standard therapy. Chest X-rays and cultures should guide antimicrobial therapy, and infections should be aggressively managed.

LIP has an insidious onset with cough and breathlessness. The chest X-ray shows widespread fine shadowing which is unresponsive to therapy. With time, and during episodes of respiratory infections, significant hypoxia may necessitate sporadic or long-term administration of supplemental oxygen. Again, parents may be able to use home oxygen therapy, given support from community nurses.

Experience with adult patients shows that the CD4 count is a sensitive indicator of disease progression, and current recommendations are that patients with CD4 counts below 200 cells/mm should be started on prophylactic therapy to prevent pneumocystis carinii pneumonia. This could take the form of trimethoprim-sulphamethoxazole or pentamidine. The latter can be given to older children who can cooperate with face masks, either in the child's home or in the GP's surgery. At present, no cure exists for HIV infection. Although much progress has been made with antiretroviral therapy, clear guidelines do not yet exist for treating children.

Immunization

The Joint Committee on Vaccination and Immunization has issued definite guidelines about the immunization of HIV seropositive children in the UK.[6]

Inactivated vaccines (diphtheria, tetanus, pertussis) should be given to all children regardless of HIV status. Live vaccines (polio, measles, mumps, rubella) are also considered safe for HIV-infected children. However, there may be some risk of complications with the use of live polio vaccination, and some clinicians may choose to use inactivated polio vaccines for the child. BCG vaccination is contraindicated in this country, in view of the risks of disseminated infection following vaccination compared with the low endemicity of tuberculosis. Because infected children's response to the vaccine may not be optimal, their antibody levels should be closely monitored following immunization, and hyperimmune globulin may have to be considered.

Hepatitis B infection is also common among injecting drug misusers and it is wise to check a woman's hepatitis B status when her child is born, and the infant given gammaglobulin and vaccine as appropriate.

The HIV-affected family

Most cases of paediatric AIDS are due to vertical transmission: about 80 per cent of children with HIV come from families where one or both parents are also infected. Social services departments have a statutory duty to investigate a family whenever it is believed that a child is at risk of neglect or abuse, and because most mothers of children with HIV have a history of drug use, or there sexual partners are drug users, the family is usually investigated, with a view to placing the child's care elsewhere. In applying child protection criteria, however, each aspect of the family's circumstances should be fully assessed and it should not be automatically assumed that drug-using parents cannot care for their children. The reasons for drug use are complex, and may arise from family stress. Decisions must be governed by factors that are in the child's best interests and, as long as the drug use does not take precedence over the child's needs, it is often best for both child and mother (or parents) to remain together.

In some families, more than one child is infected, which makes additional stresses on family resources. Drug use may have alienated the extended family who will be unavailable for support or child care. If they are involved, grandparents will also have to cope with HIV infection in more than one grandchild, as well as mourn the loss of younger generations from AIDS.

The stigma of AIDS

Few other words evoke the feelings of fear, panic and hysteria that 'AIDS' does. The labelling of 'risk groups' has led to the disease being thought of as only occurring in socially disenfranchised populations such as homosexuals and drug addicts. Hearing the diagnosis of AIDS or HIV infection in a child precipitates feelings of shock, disbelief and guilt in the parents, and denial in one form or another is a common response. This may sometimes hinder parents' ability to cope with the reality of the diagnosis. Though not all families respond in the same way, it is important to bear in mind that initial intervention by the doctor, health visitor or social worker will have to focus on ways to alleviate the impact of the diagnosis. Many parents may opt not to disclose the diagnosis to other members of the family, and this can limit the potential sources of practical and emotional support. In the absence of support from extended family, medical, nursing or social work personnel often find that they need to act in an advocacy role for the child and family. This can range from obtaining benefits for the child to helping parents integrate the child into school.

Integration into the community

Sometimes a mother's or father's continued drug use may lead to inconsistent child care, or ill-health may preclude them from providing care for the child; this means that alternative care arrangements must be found, which raises further issues.[7] All child carers (foster parents, day-carers, nursery nurses, community carers) should receive in-service training on HIV infection, with particular emphasis on the known routes of transmission of the virus and the practical aspects of looking after children with HIV infection. Because it is not always possible to identify all infected children, a stress on improving standards of personal hygiene will greatly reduce chances of virus transmission. Training in the care of children known to have HIV must address health care issues, e.g. symptoms that demand prompt medical attention.

If stringent standards of hygiene are applied universally in all child care establishments, there is no reason not to follow full integration of HIV-infected children into day-care facilities, nurseries or schools, if the child's health permits.[8]

Decisions about where to place children who are incontinent or have behavioural problems (biting) should be made on an individual basis. With the parents' consent, it is advisable to have a multidisciplinary meeting involving medical and education staff to discuss the best placement for the child, which may involve facilities for special educational needs. Similar requirements are also necessary for children whose health may not permit mainstream education. Clear infection control guidelines are provided for school staff[8,9] who should also seek advice and support from the school health team. There is a need for a policy in schools that should indicate who should authorize the sharing of information and by whom. At all times, it is important to ask: Who *needs* to know about the HIV-infected child and why?

Telling the child

As with all chronic illnesses, parents may be at a loss to know how, what and whether to disclose the diagnosis to the child. The amount and quality of information they decide to give will obviously depend on the maturity of the child. When a child is subjected to the rigours of medical intervention, some explanation ought to be given and most parents have their way of doing so. Talking to children about their condition and anticipating their questions often reduces their anxiety; in some instances, play therapy is useful in allowing children to act out fears and fantasies.

The adolescent with HIV infection has needs not always recognized by current medical or social work practice. In this country, most adolescents with HIV infections are haemophiliacs, although some will be infected as a result of sexual contact or injecting drug use. The normal vulnerability of adolescence is compounded by the secrecy of their disease, and the difficulties imposed by HIV on sexual relationships. It is good for an infected adolescent to have a particular person identified to talk to about matters such as the prevention of infection in others, relationships and their disease. Whoever is identified for this role must be prepared to give repeated support and help when requested. Most adolescents will also wish to be part of the decision-making team on issues regarding disease management, including a possible decision not to continue with therapeutic intervention.

Terminal illness

Throughout the course of the illness, the primary focus for community health workers is on helping the families to come to terms with and to cope with HIV infection in the child. But with each hospital admission comes the growing awareness of a terminal illness, and feelings of guilt, anger, grief and denial will re-emerge. There may be the added pain of the secrecy of AIDS. Parents have to decide whether they wish to nurse the child at home, in a hospice or in hospital. Children whose parents have already died from AIDS may be placed in foster care, and social work departments need to develop clear policies on the care of terminally ill children and how to support foster parents in this care.

A primary concern of parents is that their child be free from pain. Parents need to be part of any decisions made during the final stages of the child's life, and, if the child is at home, professionals should keep regular contact with them through home visits or telephone calls, to let the families know that help is still available.

The paediatric counselling and screening clinic

Because so little is known about the natural history of HIV infection in children, and as their care and management present so many challenges, we established a clinic in Edinburgh in January 1986 to monitor all infants born to HIV-infected women.[10] This clinic is one of 10 centres participating in a

European Collaborative Study to evaluate the risk of materno-fetal transmission of HIV.[11] The progress and treatment of all participating children are monitored.

The paediatric clinic is held in conjunction with an adult HIV screening and counselling clinic. It is staffed by a consultant paediatrician with an interest in community child health, a health visitor and a paediatric registrar. The majority of referrals are from the adult clinic who are already monitoring the health of many HIV positive women. Other referrals are from antenatal clinics throughout the city, GPs, neonatal and general paediatricians, health visitors and social workers.

Pregnant women with HIV often want advice about the likelihood of passing on the virus to the child, and about what sort of outlook a child with HIV has, so one of the paediatricians from the clinic usually meets the woman in the antenatal period to discuss these issues. Some women decide to terminate their pregnancy, but if a woman decides to have the child, the purpose and nature of monitoring the child's health is described, and she is asked for permission to include the child in the study. One of the paediatricians is also present at delivery to obtain cord blood and to examine the infant. Future visits are then arranged, either at the clinic or at home.

The clinic's model is that of a family clinic, and children are seen along with their parent(s); this extends to visits to the family's home. There is close liaison between medical staff responsible for parent's health care and paediatric staff, which has resulted in good communication on all aspects of the care of the family as a whole. The surveillance procedure is outlined in

Table 1 Support for HIV-infected families from the paediatric counselling and screening clinic, Edinburgh

In the antenatal period
● Counselling on advisability of continued pregnancy
● Discuss effects of transmission from mother to child
● Offer follow-up of mother and child
● Support throughout pregnancy

Follow-up of child
● Regular review for growth, development and signs of HIV infection
● Monitoring of laboratory tests
● Immunization
● Discuss child care issues
● Liaise with social work and education staff, as necessary

At every visit, the parent's health and use of drugs should be enquired into, and if necessary, referral made to
● Adult physician
● Drug rehabilitation programme
● Social work department on child care, housing or financial matters
● Voluntary agencies/self-help groups

Table 1. In-patient facilities are available at the Infectious Diseases Unit of the City Hospital in Edinburgh, where admission is under the care of the consultant paediatrician; thus continuity of care is maintained.

Conclusion

The lack of a definitive cure for HIV infection does not imply that nothing can be done to help HIV-affected families. Children with HIV infection and their families present tremendous and complex challenges to medical, nursing, social work and education professionals as well as members of voluntary agencies. The multiple problems encountered when dealing with an HIV-infected child demands a high degree of collaboration between hospital and community services, to provide a service which is well co-ordinated and comprehensive.

References

1 Peutherer, J. F., Edmond, E., Simmonds, P., Dickson, J. D. and Bath, G. E. (1985). HTLV III antibody in Edinburgh drug addicts. *Lancet*, ii, 1129–30.
2 Robertson, J. R., Bucknall, A. B. V., Welsby, P. D., Roberts, J. J. K., Inglis, J. M., Peutherer, J. F. and Brettle, R. P. (1986). An epidemic of AIDS related virus (HTLV III/LAV) infection amongst intravenous drug abusers in a Scottish general practice. *British Medical Journal*, **292**, 527–30.
3 Brettle, R. P., Bissett, K., Burns, S., Davidson, J., Davidson, S. J., Gray, J. M. N., Inglis, J. M., Lees, J. S. and Mok, J. (1987). Human immunodeficiency virus and drug misuse: The Edinburgh experience. *British Medical Journal*, **295**, 421–4.
4 Johnstone, F. D., MacCallum, L., Brettle, R., Inglis, J. M. and Peutherer, J. F. (1988). Does infection with HIV affect the outcome of pregnancy? *British Medical Journal*, **296**, 467.
5 Hague, R. A., Yap, P. L., Mok, J. Y. Q., Eden, O. B., Coutts, N. A., Watson, J. G., Hargreaves, F. D. and Whitelas, J. M. (1989). Intravenous immunoglobulin in HIV infection. Evidence for the efficacy of treatment. *Archives of Disease in Childhood*, **64**, 1146–50.
6 Joint Committee on Vaccination and Immunization. Department of Health and Social Security, Welsh Office, Scottish Home and Health Department (1988). *Immunisation against Infectious Disease*. London, HMSO.
7 Batty, D. (ed.) (1987). *The Implications of AIDS for Children in Care*. Discussion Series 9. London, British Agencies for Adoption and Fostering.
8 Department of Education and Science and Welsh Office (1986). *Children at School and Problems Related to AIDS*. London, HMSO.
9 Scottish Education Department (1987). *AIDS – Guidance for Educational Establishments in Scotland*. Edinburgh, HMSO.
10 Mok, J. Y. Q., Hague, R. A., Taylor, R. F., Brettle, R. P., Hargreaves, F. D., Inglis, J. M. and Yap, P. L. (1989). The management of children born to human immunodeficiency virus seropositive women. *Journal of Infection*, **18**, 119–24.
11 The European Collaborative Study (1988). Mother-to-child transmission of HIV infection. *Lancet*, ii, 1039–42.

Index

morbidity—*cont'd*
 inequality in, 67
 see also illness; National Morbidity
  Study
mother and toddler groups, 57–8
mothers
 as carers, 6–7, 9–10, 18, 24–5,
  29–38, 41, 45–6, 50, 56–62, 138–9
 competence of, 6–7, 10, 16–17, 29,
  33–5, 45, 139
 concerns and vulnerabilities of, 36–8
 expertise of, 45
 feelings of inadequacy of, 34–5,
  134–6
 knowledge of, 30–32, 59–60, 138
 perceived neuroticism of, 35–8, 141
 perspectives of, 53
 responsibility of, 33–4, 55–6, 141
 self-esteem of, 18, 34–5, 134–5

National Asthma Campaign, 127, 129
National Health Service, 3–6
 see also health services; health
  professionals
National Morbidity Study, 67
nurseries, provision of, 54, 57–8
 see also mother and toddler groups

parents
 consulting behaviour of, 67–9, 71–2,
  74–6, 79–87
 decision making of, 1, 29–30, 41,
  71–2, 74–6, 86–7
 diagnosis by, 1
patients
 perspectives of, 51
 rights of, 2
perspectives
 health visitors', 53, 100
 mothers', 53–4, 100
 parents', 61–2
play areas, 49–50
 and outdoor space, 58
postnatal care, 89, 95
poverty, 50
 and links with health, 15–16, 25, 59,
  101
pregnancy, 49–50
 and antenatal care, 47–51, 92–3
 and caesarean section, 92

and delivery care, 48, 89, 92
 fasting in, 46–7, 50
 and HIV, 145, 149–50
 termination of, 149–50
prescriptions, 95–6, 98, 100–101, 121,
  124–5

qualitative methods, 30

racism, 44–5, 48–9
 in health care, 41, 50–51, 89–90
religion, 7
 Islamic, 42–3, 46–7, 89
 observance of, 42–3
 and prayer, 49
 and purdah, 48
respiratory illness, 8, 67–9, 72, 76–7,
  80–1, 86, 109, 144
 consultations for, 67–8, 75–7, 82–3
 morbidity from, 67–8

sexual abuse, 9–10, 133
 discovery of, 133, 139
 and 'good' mothering, 133, 136, 141
 and health professionals, 10, 134,
  137–9, 141–2
 and incest, 134–6, 138
 and mother-blaming, 10, 134–6
 and mother–child relationship, 133,
  136, 141
smoking, 15, 69–70, 79, 110
social class
 and breastfeeding, 107–11
 occupational, 67–8
social contacts, 42–3, 57–9
social networks, 48, 54–7
social services, 25–6, 59–60
social skills, 44–5, 57
social support, 90–91, 98, 100–101,
  147
socio-economic circumstances, *see*
  benefits; education; housing; inner-
  city areas; money; poverty; social
  class; transport; unemployment;
  work, paid
stimulation, 55–9
 and development of language, 54–6
 and development of motor skills, 56
 see also child development
symptoms, 6–7, 93–4, 97, 100, 109–10

transport, 43, 54, 69–70

unemployment, 54, 68–70, 79, 90

welfare rights 25–6, 32
work, paid, 7, 54, 90–1

and low income, 15–22
manual, 43, 69–70, 79
and mental health, 59
and women, 7, 15–17, 24, 29–30,
    57–8, 79, 90–91